Barbara Morris, R. Ph.

No More Little Old Ladies!

15 Essential & Specific
Proven Anti-Aging
Strategies for Gutsy
Women in Their
40s and 50s

(And for very, very
gutsy women in
their 60s
& beyond)

New York

No More Little Old Ladies!

by Barbara Morris, R., Ph.

This book is written as a source of information only. The information, ideas and suggestions contained in this book by no means should be considered a substitute for the advice of a qualified medical professional, who should always be consulted before beginning any new diet, exercise, procedure, or health program.

All efforts have been made to ensure the accuracy of the information contained in this book as of the date of publication. The author/publisher expressly disclaims responsibility for any adverse effects arising from the use or application of the information, ideas, and suggestions contained herein.

ISBN 978-1-60037-521-7

Library of Congress Control Number: 2008936944

Published by:

MORGAN · JAMES
THE ENTREPRENEURIAL PUBLISHER ™
www.morganjamespublishing.com

Morgan James Publishing, LLC
1225 Franklin Ave. Ste 325
Garden City, NY 11530-1693
Toll Free 800-485-4943
www.MorganJamesPublishing.com

Interior Design by:
Bonnie Bushman
bbushman@bresnan.net

In an effort to support local communities, raise awareness and funds, Morgan James Publishing donates one percent of all book sales for the life of each book to Habitat for Humanity.

Get involved today, visit

www.HelpHabitatForHumanity.org.

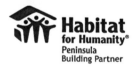

Habitat
for Humanity®
Peninsula
Building Partner

Acknowledgments

Thanks to editors Barbara McNichol and Dr. Patricia Ross for transforming the manuscript into real-world help for women in their forties and fifties who want to avoid becoming Little Old Ladies. Their insights into the "midlife mind" have been invaluable, and I am grateful for their help and expertise.

Dedication

To every young-to-midlife woman who knows "old age" is unavoidable but that being "old" is a choice and that she can choose to be ageless for the rest of her life.

Testimonials

I tell all my clients that reading your newsletter and your book is a necessity. You bring unique and essential information on aging that we do not gain from a physician or counselors, specializing in the aging field. Your pharmaceutical background and knowledge is a real blessing.

Helen Harkness, PhD,
Career Design Associates, Inc., Garland, Texas

Between what Barbara Morris knows as a pharmacist, what she knows as an antiaging coach and evangelist, and what she demonstrates in how she's living her own ageless life, her counsel is worth heeding. Read *No More Little Old Ladies!* It's full of exhilarating revelations and advice.

Mary Lloyd, CEO,
Mining Silver and author of *Bold Retirement*

Contents

Introduction

How Old Are You?

If you're in your forties, you probably don't think twice about telling someone how old you are. You may even say, "I'm forty-three," with pride, because you know you don't look or act like what you think the rest of the world thinks forty-three ought to look or act like.

If you're in your fifties, you might be a bit more reluctant to divulge your age. You hesitate because, even though you still don't think you look or act "old," and you probably don't think of yourself as "middle-aged," you're starting to realize that you may have more years behind you than ahead of you. Let's look at two scenarios:

1. If you're in your sixties and you're in good shape, you may still think of yourself as forty. You may see some definite signs that time is passing by, but because you planned well and took care of yourself mentally and physically, you probably feel and function as you did when you were forty. You deliberately don't tell anyone how old you are because you can get away with people treating you at the age they perceive you to be.

2.   However, if you're in your sixties, and you've just allowed life to happen—which most people do—you're going to start to feel old physically and mentally. You don't have enough energy. You have achy joints and stomach and digestion problems. You can't remember where you put your keys. You laugh and say, "Oh, I'm having a senior moment," and then you go on, trudging through your day and complaining about looking and feeling old.

Ladies, if you're now in your forties or fifties, you *can* have the first sixties scenario. The "getting old" part of aging is something we women constantly fear. We think that it's just part of our genetic heritage. And because the baby boomers are starting to reach middle age, there are all kinds of messages—both subtle and overt—about being okay with getting old.

How many times have you seen the second sixties scenario played out over and over on TV sitcoms and in commercials? But you know what? It doesn't have to be that way! You don't have to live a life of a "Little Old Lady." However, if you don't have the right antiaging diet and the right antiaging mind-set and lifestyle, you're going to find yourself old at sixty—the age when it all starts to catch up with you. If you're in your forties or fifties, start *now* with the antiaging regimen in this book. The longer you wait to take action, the more difficult it is to overcome the effects of aging.

How do I know? I'm seventy-nine years old. But I don't ever tell my age unless it's important because I don't look seventy-nine, and I certainly don't feel seventy-nine. Now, it's important for me to tell you my age because this is a book about helping you avoid becoming a Little Old Lady. It's a how-to guide to getting and keeping an antiaging lifestyle—and that includes not only the right regimen of diet and exercise but also a constant, vigilant watch on your attitude and mind-set about aging.

You can find a lot of books out there on aging. Aging, like cancer, is big business. But most of these books are written by people who are under sixty-five. What do they know about old age? I've been through the things that you're going to go through. I know what you need to be aware of. I am a pharmacist, and I worked until I was seventy-six. I stopped working not because it was time to retire but because it was time for a career change. I was ready to move on to bigger and better things. It was time to indulge my passion— writing and helping younger women achieve what I have. Practicing pharmacy as long as I did was the best medicine I could have ever taken. Not only did I keep a young mind-set because I was working and interacting with younger people, but I also saw the parade of old people pass by my pharmacy window every day. What I saw was sobering. It was a world I knew I didn't want to become part of.

I witnessed firsthand the senior culture in all of its aspects—the never-ending supply of pills that seniors would take for their aches and pains, the "old" lifestyle that they lived. Women much younger than I used to complain, "Barbara, I feel so old. Don't ever get old." I could never empathize with what they were feeling, mostly because I was not yet where they were in life, even though I was much older. I had yet to experience what it meant to "feel old." (I still haven't experienced what it means to "feel old.") Every time I heard the "I feel so old" lament, I used to think, "There but for the grace of God go I." Then I would vow to keep up my antiaging lifestyle.

Experience is the best teacher, and I've experienced how to avoid traditional decline. I live this stuff every day. If you are interested in finding out how I stay young, including looking and feeling young, read on. If you want to accept yourself as you are—your expanding middle, your loss of youthful vitality—that's okay. But know the consequences: you will look and feel old at sixty when you don't have to.

Little Old Lady Syndrome—It Is Avoidable

If you're in your forties or fifties, you probably aren't thinking about what it will be like to be a Little Old Lady. You even avoid thinking about it because you don't want to think about the inevitable. But you should think about it.

Like beauty, old is in the eye of the beholder. How do you think of old? Here's a simple test. Is this describing a young woman or an old woman?

- She projects energy.
- She speaks with animation.
- She moves confidently.
- She has interests beyond her immediate world.
- She listens and quickly processes and understands what she hears.
- She is aware.
- She is productive.
- She is other-oriented.
- She is not envious of other women or women who look "better."
- She values the company and friendship of people of all ages.
- She lives a vigorous, healthy lifestyle.
- She has a toned, supple body.
- She continues to grow.
- She ignores her chronological age and lives her perceived age.
- She cultivates and maintains a strong inner drive— her "inner pit bull."
- She rejects "victimhood" because it accelerates aging.
- She avoids (as one would a plague) the senior culture. (More on this in a bit.)

If you said this is a young woman, you are like too many women out there. You've been led to believe that only young women are like this. However, I know from my own experience and from helping many women like you that all these attributes can be yours as you age, no matter how chronologically old you are.

Based on my experience, I know that there are three main reasons why a woman becomes a Little Old Lady:

1.   According to the book *Successful Aging* by John W. Rowe, MD, 70 percent of the aging process is controllable through wise lifestyle choices. Only 30 percent of how we age is the result of heredity. Few women know that they have such awesome power, and they give it up by default.

2.   Of the few women who do understand that they have such astonishing power, most don't believe that it's possible to manage or else they don't see the value in attempting to manage how they age.

3.   Even those women who believe it's possible—who see the value in maintaining youthful attributes and characteristics as long as possible, and who want to control their aging process—usually don't know how to go about doing it.

Bottom line: A Little Old Lady is not about physical appearance. It's not about whether you have gray hair and wrinkles. *A Little Old Lady is a woman who has succumbed to controllable influences and the ravages of the aging process.* (I'll talk about a particularly virulent controllable influence in Strategy No. 6.)

How Do You Avoid Becoming a Little Old Lady?

It's simple yet difficult.

It's difficult because a woman who desires to manage her aging process and understands that it's possible to do so must begin at least by age forty to develop the mind-set, behaviors, constant determination, and regimen that it takes to be successful. Frankly, it involves unleashing "pit bull" willpower. You have to dig deep into your psyche to find it, and to be perfectly honest, most women can't find it because they don't try hard enough or just don't see the value in trying. But I'll bet *you* can if you are tenacious enough!

Why is it so difficult to avoid becoming a Little Old Lady? At age forty, you aren't thinking about what you want to be like or what you want your life to be like twenty-five or thirty-five years into the future. At age forty, you are thinking about all the pressing issues you have to deal with today. You have little time or inclination to think about the future. So, even with a desire to control the aging process, life usually overpowers it with concerns about the mortgage, the kids, and the career—in other words, what's happening *now*.

Then there is the reality factor. A woman at age forty looks at sixty-five- and seventy-five-year-old women who have aged traditionally. What she sees tells her that she will likely (but hopefully not!) experience the same degree of deterioration.

But here's the thing. We usually don't notice the sixty-five- and seventy-five-year-old women who have learned how to manage the aging process. We look at them and think they are younger because they typically function as they did years earlier. In addition, they look years younger, either through diet and exercise and/or the help of some cosmetic procedure.

Here's another import element: women who project an aura of youthfulness far into their older years often are "in the age closet"—by choice. And when you get to that point, you'll know what I'm talking about. This is what happens: when coworkers or friends suddenly discover the age of an older woman who appears much younger, they often exclaim "Wow! You are *that* old? Good for you!" First, who wants to hear that? And second, once your friends or coworkers know your age, something not so subtle happens. The relationship between the outed older woman and those who know the truth about her age will never be the same. She will be subject to the biases, perceptions, and expectations that others have about how a woman "that age" should be, and she will be treated accordingly.

Whereas before she would be expected to hold her own, all of a sudden she hears things like, "Here, let me help you with that" or "Be careful, don't fall!" Worse, because most people think that older people lose it as time goes on, the older woman is passed over for a promotion at work (accompanied by a lame explanation) or relegated to easy tasks that don't challenge her physically or, worse, mentally.

Thus, it's less stressful for a young "older woman" to stay in the age closet.

Obviously, women who appear younger and function as if they are younger are not yet the norm, in spite of the cliché that age sixty is the new forty. When these women do attract public attention, they are often regarded as anomalies—probably self-absorbed women who have focused excessively on staying young. News of this sort often generates disdain and/or envy and does nothing to encourage younger women to take charge of their aging process.

Here is something else that works against women making an effort to be ageless: in our society, women are increasingly encouraged to accept their bodies as they are—which often means accepting some degree of obesity or unfitness. The result is that many women at age forty have a grudging contentment with where they are.

When a woman accepts the subliminal message from society that she is okay just the way she is and doesn't have to change a thing, it leads her to not even think about what she could be twenty-five to thirty-five years down the road. On a recent TV show, out-of-shape young women stripped down to their skimpy underwear and were encouraged to love themselves as they are. Would the young women be better served if they were encouraged to take more control over their lifestyles and focus on their future well-being?

It's simple to avoid becoming a Little Old Lady if you believe it's possible and desire to manage your aging process. You must have a compelling vision of how you want to be mentally and physically twenty-five to thirty-five years into the future, and you must be willing to commit to implementing and sticking with a regimen that will make it happen.

The keywords in the previous statement are "vision" and "regimen."

Having a living, breathing vision of how you will be in twenty-five to thirty-five years is fundamental for achieving success. You have to develop in your mind's eye a detailed, moving picture of what you will be like and how you will be living in the future. Once that motion picture of your future self is firmly embedded in your mind and constantly replayed, refined, and nurtured, it will drive the choices you make about how you live your life. You will become what you focus upon and think about most consistently.

In case you missed it: *Once that moving picture of your future self is firmly embedded in your mind and constantly replayed, refined, and nurtured, it will drive the choices you make about how you live your life. You will become what you focus upon and think about most consistently.*

Holding fast to a sharp, clear, compelling vision will guide you into forming beliefs, behaviors, attitudes, and actions that will lead you to your goal. You may encounter roadblocks along the way because we are not in total control of what happens to us. Nevertheless, if you keep the living, breathing vision of your future self always in the forefront of your consciousness, you will be rewarded far beyond your expectations.

My personal vision is that of a strong, slender, healthy woman. I have been watching that vision for so long and it is so firmly embedded in my mind that when I am tempted to slack off on exercise or eat what I shouldn't, my vision appears in sharp focus and I am able to adjust my behavior to stay in sync with my vision. Don't scoff. It works for me and can work for you.

It becomes extraordinarily simple to avoid becoming a Little Old Lady when you have learned the techniques necessary to develop and live an antiaging lifestyle and you have put them into practice. In fact, it's so simple that it comes down to implementing that motion picture in your mind through a daily regimen or system.

It's like McDonald's—not their food but the way they work. They have a proven system to prepare food and run the operation that restaurants repeat in the exact same way every day. Following the system without deviation produces a desired result. Avoidance of Little Old Lady-ness is accomplished the same way. You educate yourself about how to live an antiaging lifestyle. You eat an antiaging diet, take antiaging supplements, and exercise every day. Most important, you develop a mind-set that helps you manage your aging process. It becomes so automatic and so much a part of your daily life that you don't go through the mental gymnastics of "should I or shouldn't I do it today." You know what you have to do, and you do it. When unforeseen events get in the way, you do what you have to do and get back into the regimen as quickly as possible.

Boring? Absolutely not. When you have a good antiaging regimen of diet, exercise, and strong positive thoughts, you operate at a high level of health and energy. As time goes on, intensely gratifying results appear right before your eyes. You realize that this is where you want to stay. You don't want to fall back. You understand that youth is a temporary gift and keeping youthful attributes takes effort.

If you're in your forties or fifties and you work to get and stay in shape, you can enjoy superior health now. The result is extremely liberating and motivating, but there is one drawback: you get to appreciate the *phenomenal* payoff, the true value of all your hard work, only when you have lived long enough.

At age seventy-nine, I feel and function as I did when I was forty. I credit this to the antiaging lifestyle I've led and continue to lead. My heart aches when I see my peers who have become Little Old Ladies, and it is because of them that I am compelled to write this book.

I've said it before, and I'll say it again. The Little Old Lady syndrome has nothing to do with wrinkles or gray hair. That's the last thing a woman who wants to control her aging process worries about. Wrinkles can be eliminated or diminished cosmetically, and hair color can be changed in forty-five minutes or less. It's the other stuff that's critically important—including but not limited to having a vision, knowing it's possible to achieve it, and finding the pit bull determination to make it happen.

Got it? Great! Now let's get on with discovering what it takes to avoid becoming a Little Old Lady.

Strategy No. 1:

Know Thy Enemy

Why Most Get "Old" and Few Stay Ageless

W hy do certain people who are the same age appear young longer than others? Is it just luck or good genes? The answer is that it's both. But there is more to it than that. Those who appear significantly younger than their age have a secret. They purposefully decide to not be old. It's not really a secret, of course, but it may as well be because so few women understand it.

Before we go further, I want to answer a question that I bet some of you are thinking. While you like what I've said up to this point—that you can manage the aging process—the little doubting voice in your head that always lurks around might be saying, "Barbara, aren't you suffering a prolonged middle-age crisis?" My answer is an emphatic *no*.

Let's talk about the definition of middle age. What does it mean to you? It used to be that age forty was considered middle age, but forty isn't middle age anymore. In the past century, the life span has increased by thirty years years. In 1900, the life expectancy was 47.3 years. According to the Centers for Disease Control and Prevention (CDC), in 2002 that number had risen to 77.3 years. That being true, how do we now define middle age?

We do it by recognizing that a longer lifespan has given us two midlife periods. The first midlife is forty to sixty. The second midlife is sixty to eighty. (This is according to futurist author Helen Harkness, and I'll discuss this in greater detail in Strategy No. 6.) Based on my chronological age and my longer life expectation, I am now in my second midlife and I intend to stay there because I know what it takes. So the question, "Barbara, aren't you suffering a prolonged middle-age crisis?" is meaningless. Staying ageless is about living your perceived age, and while we do age chronologically, we have the ability to not feel and behave old—and isn't that what we would all like to do? My perceived age is forty (even though I am in my second midlife), and that's the way I live. You can do it, too. I hope that with all of your being you will decide not to be old. I want to stress again: aging is inevitable; being old is a choice.

What Usually Happens

This is what all of you are actually up against. Right now you are either somewhere right before or right at the make-or-break point of the aging process. We can easily divide this process into two parts: before age fifty and after age fifty. Until you are forty or more, you don't think much about how you are aging. Am I right? Constantly feeling youthful keeps you from dwelling too much on thoughts about getting old. You have more important things to worry about.

Something about youth is so devious, so tricky, and so deceitful—or so it seems. You look in the mirror every day, and nothing seems to change. You think you look the same as you did yesterday, last week, last month. You say, perhaps with pride, "I'm doing well for my age." That's how youth cons you into thinking that you don't have to do anything to keep your own youthfulness around.

But youth can't be devious; it doesn't have that capacity. It simply does what it is designed to do—that is, it gives you about fifty good, vibrant, visually attractive, healthy years. Then it turns you over to your human nature, or what I call your "existence manager," whose job is to lead you down the path to your inevitable destination: death.

Around age forty, you probably do begin to notice subtle changes in your appearance: wrinkles, weight gain, gray hair. You may feel advancing age in your bones. Minor health issues might begin to surface and occupy your thoughts to some extent. These are symptoms of aging, but like minor symptoms of a cold, you ignore them. You continue to take life as it comes, your youthfulness still highly evident.

You still see what you perceive as youth in the mirror every day, even though it is actually slipping away imperceptibly before your eyes. And the changes you *can* see aren't extreme enough to make you do anything to try to stop them. A little pudgier around the waist? A bit of stiffness or an achiness now and then? You justify living with what you see and feel because, really, it's not so bad.

On an awareness scale of one to ten, with ten being most aware of what's happening with your body, your level of awareness is about a two. And that is exactly the problem.

Because you know that there is a problem—slight, but present nonetheless—you do little things with makeup to disguise signs of advancing age. But that's about it. That increasing girth around the middle? You agonize over it a bit and vow to go on a diet, but in the meantime you cover the bulge with a big shirt. Or maybe you won't cover it. As I've mentioned already, we've been trained to accept and feel comfortable with our bodies as they are. After all, maybe it's just five pounds of fat that you'll easily shed when you really put your mind to it. Here's the problem: the coverup of little things furthers your self-deception. If it bothers you, then you hide the evidence to convince yourself that you're not aging so badly. When you ignore and shrug off the little stuff, when you let small, correctable things slip by, you set yourself up to accept and overlook the bigger changes that are aging you.

As you progress into your fifties and begin to notice more pronounced, middle-aged signs of physical decline, you still don't give much thought to how you're changing. You still have youthful energy and interests. You probably feel good in spite of the little aches and pains that nag at you. And you continue to live life as it comes because concerns of the day still dominate your thinking.

At this point, youth has deceived you into thinking that this feeling-good time will stick around a lot longer. You continue to cover up or ignore signs of aging and declare you are satisfied with the result. After all, you still look young enough. And the weight gain? You've gained five more pounds. To make yourself feel better, you promise to eat better and exercise and you buy a size larger jeans—just for now. You begin to diet in earnest. You rationalize that you can fit into the smaller jeans after the weight comes off. The diet leaves you hungry and cranky, so you give it up after a couple of days. The weight never comes off.

When you were just five pounds overweight was the golden opportunity to nip the weight gain in the bud. But you didn't, and that's when you started to give up control of your body and your aging process. What you didn't know then was that *you were letting go.* So your solution to the problem actually created more problems because you were beginning to feel resigned to how you were changing.

As the process of letting go continues, your existence manager thumbs its nose at your apathy and pulls you another step closer to the inevitable outcome: the end of your existence. You don't want to give in to the push and pull of your existence manager, but you don't know how to stop it. As your resignation deepens, your body continues to morph into a midlife muddle and your mind-set settles into comfortable "middle-age think" You resolve to recapture waning or lost youthful attributes, but by that time major damage may have been done. Your existence manager— the lure toward life's end—has taken over, doing what it's supposed to do. You begrudgingly accept this path to oldness, i.e., inevitable decline. You're not happy, but what can you do? Certainly, you can improve as long as you live and breathe, but it's difficult to get back what has been lost. The longer you wait to take corrective action, the more difficult it is. An aging body unaccustomed to being pushed around resists change.

As time passes and you approach your sixties, your feelings of resignation continue to deepen. After all, everyone else your age, with few exceptions, looks and feels the way you do. So you go with the flow. You accept subliminal "you are getting old" messages from society. In a creeping way, you start to think of yourself as a "senior." Slowly, and perhaps without even realizing it, you step into the senior culture that your existence manager embraces. But beware: *the senior culture is the speedway to your final destination.* I talk about it specifically in Strategy No. 6.

Strategy No. 2:
Discover and Use Your Ultimate Power Tool

Be Aware!

I have discovered many secrets for controlling or managing the aging process. The most important secret, as I said in Strategy No. 1, is to consciously decide to be young, if not physically, then at least mentally. From that decision, I found the ultimate personal "power tool" to keep me young: *I maintain an ongoing awareness of how I am changing mentally and physically.* You can't control or manage what you don't notice.

Because it has become acceptable to accept ourselves just the way we are, we've been given the okay to stick our heads in the sand and pretend that all those signs of aging are just not there. However, I have found that if I remain alert to and aware of the changes in my physical appearance and mental attitude, I can stop or at least try to mitigate what I can control.

For example, I am constantly aware of signs that I may be adopting "old thinking." I listen to old people and try not to emulate their "old" speech and habits, which are outcomes of controllable old thinking. For example, I may hear, "I'm having a bad day. I can't remember where I put my keys. I must be getting old." Is such a declaration a fact or just habitual old thinking? Wouldn't it be just as easy to say, "This is a great day. I am feeling super. I *will* remember where I put my keys."

You may be feeling like crap (sorry for being crude, but you know what I mean, don't you?), but you know you have the power to decide how you say you feel. You can "fake it till you make it." Many times I have laughed at myself when I'm in a bit of a funk about where I put something, and while in the process of faking it, I feel better—no kidding. You may not remember where you put your misplaced item right away, but the endorphins that have been released in your brain as a result of positive self-talk will eventually help soothe you and enable you to recall where you left the missing item. Try it. It works for me—sooner or later.

Another old behavior I try to avoid is telling my age, especially when it serves no purpose. On a TV home shopping show, I watched two women call in with product testimonials and right off they told their ages—seventy-six and seventy-eight. Their ages had no relevance to anything. Furthermore, they didn't have to tell their ages because the sound of their voices gave them away. (You *can* control the sound of your voice as you age. Stay aware of the pitch and tone and how much energy you project. Put a smile and youthful enthusiasm into your speech.)

What *do* you say when people blurt out their ages for no apparent reason? It's embarrassing, and it puts you on the spot. In the previous instance, the show host responded with "Congratulations!" It's a silly reply, but there isn't much else he could have said. Is it appropriate to congratulate someone for being lucky enough to live so long? The problem is, by telling people your age, you are thinking old. Think about it. Young people do not advertise their ages. Their youth is obvious, and the "how old" aspect of life has little meaning to them.

As I've aged chronologically, I've become very aware that old people like to tell their ages because it often results in a comment such as "You look great for your age" or "You don't look your age." It's a dead giveaway that they are looking for compliments, and it's old behavior. As I told you in the introduction, I refrain from telling my age unless it serves a purpose. I don't like to see my age in print, and I do not like to hear the sound of my voice reinforcing what I am trying to ignore! I try to live my perceived age, which is forty, but I *am* seventy-nine. I am consciously making a choice to not see or hear my age so that my mind's computer doesn't get confused. There is a part of the mind that interprets everything we do or say literally, so when I must tell how young I am, I deliberately flush the reference to my chronological age as quickly as possible.

There is another old behavior that some older women tend to engage in: they get to a point in life where they think others are curious about them, and they feel obligated to tell everyone about their past—especially the unsavory parts.

For example, Barbara Walters recently revealed that thirty years ago she had an affair with a married U.S. senator.

The cad in question, Senator Edward Brooke, is still alive. To make matters worse, he has remarried and presumably his new wife had been unaware of the affair until Barbara blabbed. The wife has since become a victim of Barbara's need for public catharsis. Thankfully, Brooke had enough class not to comment on Barbara's revelation.

It appears that Barbara has become a typical Little Old Lady. She doesn't look like what most of us would consider a Little Old Lady, but remember that appearance is not what makes a woman a Little Old Lady. Barbara, at seventy-something, seems to have lost the ability to think rationally—one of the hallmarks of a Little Old Lady in the process of decline. I think the part of the brain that helps manage behavior turns to concrete in some older individuals. Old people sometimes get so far out of touch with reality and so deeply into themselves that they lose awareness of what is acceptable thinking and behavior.

I know that times have changed. But for the most part, what was not acceptable behavior thirty years ago is still not acceptable. However, we have become accustomed to bad behavior and often accept it with a "so what" attitude. We have lost our sense of moral outrage. I believe that an older woman with half a brain left in her head should not air her dirty linen in public—for any reason. It's called preserving what may be left of one's self-respect. If Barbara felt a need to clear her conscience, she could have talked privately to her rabbi or a counselor.

She didn't have to embarrass herself or create pain for Brooke's new wife, nor did she have to cause legions of women to feel embarrassed and ashamed for her. In effect, by behaving like a mindless, immature Hollywood teenager, she devalued not only herself but also the status of all older women in the eyes of the world. No wonder many people often accuse older people of having lost their minds. Clearly, in this instance, Barbara lost it, and her thoughtless behavior reflects negatively on all older women.

Young women who have had their innate sense of shame and self-respect decimated by popular culture think nothing of publicly exposing themselves in every conceivable manner. I pity them. However, older women who still have their wits about them are aware of the ramifications of unacceptable behavior and so keep their sins to themselves.

The lesson to be learned from the Walters fiasco is to sharpen your awareness of the quality and purpose of your behavior and to better take charge of how you're managing changes in your life. Maintaining awareness of change is difficult for most people. I think the reason for this may be that the pull of our human nature or existence manager, whose job it is to lead us to our final destination, is stronger than our good intentions. However, in spite of that constant pull to the finish line, you *do* have the ability to stay aware of how you are changing. And if you do maintain awareness and act on what you're aware of, you're light-years ahead of your peers who aren't attentive to their mental and physical changes.

I've already mentioned it but it bears mentioning again because it's so important: when you combine the power of an embedded vision in your mind of the way you want to be in twenty-five years along with a constant state of awareness of how you are changing, it is dynamite. It puts you in charge of your future in a way that's difficult to imagine. Unfortunately, you get to realize the power of this dynamic duo of awareness of change and visualization only when you are sixty-five, seventy-five, and beyond. But what a payoff when you get there!

By age ten, I knew I never wanted to be old. I felt it to the core of my being, and I still feel it. I didn't like old people because they always seemed to be sick and complaining. (My mother was my role model in that respect.) I saw a photo in the *Ladies Home Journal* of a pretty young woman, and I decided I always wanted to look like her. I didn't know how I was going to do it; I just knew I could and would. That picture is just as sharp and clear in my mind today as it was when I was ten. It was and remains highly motivating. By the time I was thirty, I knew instinctively about things I'd have to do to make the image in my mind come to life. No voices in my head told me what to do; I just knew. I also understood that what I put into my body and what I did to my body and my mind would determine whether I'd reach my goal.

Since you're way past ten years old, here's what I suggest you do now to create your awareness of your ideal self at sixty-five or older. No matter how old you are now, develop a detailed mental picture ("future knowing") of what you want to be like and what you want your life to be like in twenty-five years. See your life clearly and describe yourself specifically:

• What do you look like?

• How do you feel?

• How are you living?

As you create your ideal self, become committed to your vision. Having a clear, compelling vision will influence every lifestyle choice you will make and will result in huge youth dividends later in life. I will remind you of this more than once! See how you can tap into the power of having a clear vision of your preferred future. Make it a self-fulfilling prophecy. Picture yourself as a healthy, dynamic young woman. Visualize your future self as you are today or as you choose to be. By keeping that picture fixed in your memory, *in the forefront of your consciousness,* and by making a commitment to achieving it, you'll absolutely make lifestyle choices that will bring that picture to fruition.

Once you have created a full picture of your ideal self, take stock of where you currently are physically and mentally. How aware are you of how you are living and what changes are happening to you? For example, do you abuse your mind and body with food, alcohol, drugs, or behaviors that disrespect or devalue them? If so, has your body become out of shape? Do you feel depressed and lack energy? What will you do about it? How will you manage how you are changing?

In what other ways do you see change happening— change that you can control? Does your face project an angry or stressed appearance? If so, you look that way for a reason. It's nothing more than a reflection of how you are living your life and what's going on in your head. Stress is aging. As author Mary Lloyd describes in her book, *Bold Retirement*, "Whenever we assume stress is external and we can't do anything about it, we make ourselves victims. Being a victim is hard on the body and harder on the spirit. That's why victims tend to look older than they are. Same deal with stress. Have you ever caught a glimpse of yourself in the mirror when you were stressed? Who's that grumpy old person scowling back?"

You can take charge of stress. You have the power to turn things around. One of the easiest ways to do it is to deliberately develop an "attitude of gratitude" about everything that happens to you—even the "bad" things; more often than not you may discover later—often much later—that you have become a better person or that your life has changed for the better because you survived the ordeal or inconvenience. For example, when I'm in a hurry driving and traffic slows me down, I replace the negative thoughts about what's happening with an expression of gratitude. Perhaps sitting at that traffic light or in traffic is just where I'm supposed to be to avoid something worse down the road at that time.

Again, stay aware of changes. Visualize the person you want to become and the life you want to have. You can choose to embed in your mind new experiences and images because your mind accepts as real whatever pictures you give it. Furthermore, your mind will use those pictures to create your outer reality. It's not silly or new-age thinking. It's simply the way it works.

You are what you say you are, and you become
what you think about most consistently.
It's an unavoidable phenomenon.

Because of my compelling vision, which has always been in the forefront of my consciousness, and my awareness of change and ability to manage it, I have achieved my goal. Have I become the young woman I saw in the *Ladies Home Journal* years ago? Of course not. I don't look exactly like her, but I look enough like her that I feel satisfied my vision has served me well. And one more thing: I make sure my vision remains clear because I'm a work in progress—and so are you!

Take Advantage of Your 70 Percent

Again, the most effective power tool you have in your antiaging tool kit is to stay persistently aware of how you are changing, so that you can consciously manage the controllable aspects of your aging process.

In the book *Successful Aging*, Dr. John W. Rowe and Robert L. Kahn explain that with rare exceptions, only about 30 percent of physical aging can be blamed on the genes and only about half of the changes in mental function with aging are genetic. If it is so that only 30 percent of physical aging is the result of your genetic makeup, that means that 70 percent is open to your control. Think about it. That's a lot of power to have in your hands. How do you use that power?

Be one of the few people who understand the importance of having perpetual awareness of change. Be one of the few who realizes that you have control over 70 percent of the aging process. Be one of the very few who has a mental picture of your preferred future. Be one of the very few who possesses the will to achieve the possible. Here's how you do it:

- Learn about the benefits of attempting to remain ageless as long as possible. (That's why you're reading this!)

- Decide to have the vision to see your future, and never underestimate the value and power of that vision.

- Believe that it's possible to manage your aging process. Intend to do it, and carry out your intent consistently on a daily basis.

- Decide to have the will to do it. You have the power of free will. Use it to your advantage.

- Decide to have the desire to want to control or manage your aging process; your youthful, dynamic, independent older years begin with your desire today.

- Decide to have the passion to take action, knowing that you will experience a phenomenal payoff in your later years.

That's it. Right now, I want you to stop and think about the aforementioned concepts. Adopt them. Make them part of your everyday thinking. Putting them into practice in your daily life does require pit bull determination. But you have it in you to do it if you really want to!

Let me clarify what I mean by "pit bull determination." We are all born with two vital elements: a survival instinct and an existence manager. I choose to call my survival instinct my inner pit bull. (I've even given mine a name— it's a "he," and his name is Rocky.) We each have an inner pit bull, but we are all different. Some have a strong pit bull instinct, while others are less driven. If you have a tough, fierce inner pit bull, it will be easier for you to take the steps necessary to manage your aging process. And make no mistake—you can develop inner toughness because we are all capable of making choices about how we think and live. Remember that 70 percent control we have over the aging process.

This brings us to the existence manager—the "thing" we are born with whose job is to drive us to the finish line. (I've given mine a name—it's a "she," and her name is Jezebel.) With a tough inner pit bull, you can manage your existence manager and potentially add years of healthy, productive living to your life. But be aware that there will always be a constant struggle between your inner pit bull and your existence manager.

For example, my inner pit bull Rocky and my existence manager Jezebel fight for dominance all the time. This is how the struggle goes: After dinner, rather than exercise, I'd much prefer to sit on the sofa and watch *Wheel of Fortune* and *Jeopardy*. When I'm tempted in this way, I hear Rocky loud and clear: "Barbara, get on that treadmill, woman!" And that's what I do 99 percent of the time. If I don't, Rocky, well-trained beast that he is, keeps snarling and I do what I have to do to shut him up. However, all the while Rocky is snarling, Jezebel is whispering in my ear: "It's okay, Barbara. You can sit. You deserve some rest. Don't listen to that vile, ugly dog."

The point is that I have the capacity to make choices. And when I make a positive choice, it's because Rocky has won the argument. Train *your* inner pit bull, and put him in charge! (If you have a female inner pit bull, don't cut her any slack. Make her work to keep you ageless. And if you have a male existence manager, don't allow him to charm you into doing his bidding!)

Look around you at those who have aged traditionally and exist in various stages of decline. What you see is what our culture considers normal aging. Early on these people didn't control 70 percent of the aging process by being determined and making wise lifestyle choices. Either they didn't know or didn't believe they possessed the power or ability, or *they didn't try!* They just lived life as it came.

You don't have to join the ranks of those who fail to be aware of and manage how they are changing. They will age traditionally, but you don't have to. You can cultivate a vision of your desired future—and achieve it—by using workable strategies and a system for managed aging. I guarantee that you'll develop them with the help of this book. So keep reading!

Strategy No. 3:

Live with Your Lights On

You're Alive, so Glow It!

There's one thing I've noticed about the aging process that's seldom (if ever) discussed: as time goes on, the inner spark that glows brightly when you're young—that hallmark of youth—gradually dims. By the time you are at midlife or even earlier, that spark is often gone. However, by simply managing your mind and body properly, you can significantly slow the tamping down of that spark of youth. You can hold on to it far longer than you may think.

Recognize Decline in Your Life Force

Just as I cautioned you to be aware of your "old thinking," you need to be aware of when your glow starts to fade. Have you ever looked in the mirror, especially when you didn't feel good or were tired, and thought, "I look old." You're tired, and so everything—including your hair—looks tired. The next time that happens, notice how your eyes look— not the skin around them, but the brightness and shine. Is it faded or gone? Notice how the rest of your face looks. If it also looks drained and without color, you'll get an idea of what you'll look like not once in a while when you're tired but most of the time in twenty-five years—if you don't do something about it now.

When the spark in your eyes dims and the color in your face fades, it is a sign that the process of "letting go" is taking place. (I spoke about letting go earlier.) Know that this has nothing to do with the passage of time. Rather, it's because you're ceasing to give off energy. Why does this happen? It can be because you've lost your passion for life, which might be the result of depression or other disease process. It can also occur just from not maintaining awareness of how you're changing.

Of all possible reasons for the decline of the spark of the life force, I believe that traditional retirement plays a significant role if a person's health is generally good. Now I know that most of you probably haven't started to seriously think about retirement; you're building your investment portfolio and putting money into your 401Ks, but that's about the extent of it. I bet you haven't given a thought to what retirement is actually going to be like. If you aren't aware of what really happens after retirement, you need to know now.

When people enter traditional retirement, their world usually narrows and their mental and physical systems atrophy. Not right away, of course. Often, a retiree spends the first couple of years after retirement traveling and doing other activities she may have waited most of her life to do. She still has a zest for life. But eventually, the "settling down" period sets in.

I've seen this with old people at the pharmacy. They've played all the tennis they are ever going to play because arthritis has become an issue. They've taken as many long trips as they are ever going to take because it's just too tiring or expensive. More severe health problems have surfaced.

Not only are they no longer as physically active, they are no longer in touch with as many folks or as many different kinds of people as they once were. They lose the stimulation they once received through regular exchanges with others. It's a gradual process they are not even aware of most of the time. The people they stay in touch with—from the office, from the gym, from the club—gradually realize they no longer have much in common with the retirees, and the friendships eventually fall by the wayside.

Sooner or later, who populates the retiree's world? For the most part it's those in the senior culture—people of similar age and circumstances whose life forces are similarly declining. These relationships are deadly because we tend to take on the characteristics and behaviors of those we associate with most often. (I delve much further into the senior culture in Strategy No. 6.)

Then, as health problems increase, people tend to become closed in more often. A good part of the day often revolves around doctor visits and maintenance duties—burdens that get in the way of the life-affirming activities that are essential to keeping the spark alive. Constant concerns about "my problems" become paramount, even morphing into dependent, childlike behavior. The retirees increasingly rely on others for help with simple tasks such as putting on shoes or clothing. By its very nature, chronic dependence helps extinguish the spark because the dwindling life force is traded for the high-energy life force of others.

Keep Your Spark Alive

A vibrant life force and an accompanying superior quality of life can extend far beyond traditional midlife—beyond what most people expect or experience. You can achieve that by focusing on what's happening with your mind and body today—staying persistently aware of how you're changing and managing your changes to the extent you can.

I cannot stress this enough. Work to keep your inner spark firing on all cylinders. Do not willingly hand it over to others in exchange for dependence, and do not hand it over to your existence manager whose job is to take you to the end of life.

Try this: deliberately project the life force within you. Right now, stop and look at yourself in a mirror. As you look at yourself, consciously turn on the youthful light in your eyes. Pretty amazing, isn't it? If you have to think of something pleasant to generate the sparkle, then do it. When you do it often enough, it becomes easy and automatic. Turn up the corners of your mouth at the same time. Guess what? Through this process you are liberating feel-good endorphins in your brain. Do you understand what you've just done? You've made a positive, life-affirming choice! What's more, when you smile and feel good, your skin looks better.

Develop the habit that when you speak you deliberately turn on the sparkle in your eyes. Do it especially when you are speaking on the phone. I do it and am often told how young I sound. Smile broadly. Be intentionally animated. You will find that this all comes easily and effortlessly on some days. But I want you to practice for those future dark days when everything is conspiring against you keeping that spark. So when you feel down or especially when you don't feel like doing this exercise, do it anyway. You will give off energy and generate endorphins that will make you feel happier, more attractive, more youthful, more interesting, and more alive.

Practice becoming an energy-generating machine. Get in the habit of having an enigmatic Mona Lisa smile on your face as often as you can think to do it. It will automatically make your eyes light up. When the corners of your mouth are turned up in a smile, not only does your face look better, you are also generating energy. Generating and emitting energy begets more energy. Young people do it unconsciously; it's part of the "youth package" you get at birth. The wonderful thing is that you don't have to give up that gift—but you do have to make an effort to keep it. Deliberately generating energy defies the existence manager that is trying to drain the life force out of you. You can learn to maintain the glow of youth!

Watch Your Language, Lady!

You Are What You Say You Are

Part of having a strong, flexible mind is having the ability to question the status quo. Staying ageless means that you are willing and able to challenge and change your own outdated social and traditional attitudes, beliefs, and behaviors that promote oldness. Most of us inherit at least some of our "old attitude" baggage from our families. For example, your mother or grandmother may have worn "sensible shoes"—and never the white kind after Labor Day. White, sensible shoes are ugly, but you wear them anyway because that's what you're supposed to do, right? It's family and social tradition!

I've also seen older daughters and their moms wearing the same dowdy housedresses when out shopping. Old, dowdy housedresses might be really comfortable and might hide your ever-expanding middle, but a young person wouldn't be caught dead in one of those dresses. Just because your "old" mother wears them doesn't mean that you should continue the family tradition. This is not meant to disparage family ties and traditions, but it is important to know when to end the secondhand aging behaviors.

You will be happy you did, and I promise you won't feel disloyalty to your family!

The same goes for all those "old" statements we make. When you forget something, lose something, or drop something, do you exclaim, "I must be getting old"? Do you say it because you heard your mother say it while you were growing up?

I can't count the number of times my mother would say, when wanting to try something new or different, "If only I were ten years younger." If you heard that as a child, you may now feel at age forty that you are too old to start a new business. Family hand-me-down mind-sets are powerful, so think carefully about the origins of your "I'm too old" self-talk.

What you say to yourself is very powerful. Even though you don't think that your mind is recording what you say, it is, and you act on what you say. What you're always saying about getting old is exactly what you will manifest in your life.

Say No to "Senior Moments"

It's hard, however, to watch what you say about being old when our whole culture is rigged. Family influence is not the only culprit. "Oldness" chatter is all around us. For example, as my husband was enjoying the sports page of the newspaper he started to laugh. "Can you believe it? San Diego Padre Greg Maddux fell off the mound while pitching and blamed it on having senior moment!" Is Maddux an old geezer who should have retired long ago? Hardly. Maddux is forty-two,and from my perspective, that makes him a boy.

Guess what? Declaring that you're having a senior moment when you make a simple mistake isn't cute. It isn't endearing. It is aging. Remember the discussion earlier about your mind and how you can choose to implant new experiences, attitudes, and beliefs in it to support any direction you choose to take? As I suggested previously, every self-deprecating remark you think or say aloud goes right into your mind's computer in a file labeled "things I want to happen." I call the mind a computer because that's exactly the way it works. The computer on your desktop is your servant. It knows nothing except what you put into it. In the same way, your mind is your servant. It does its best to accomplish what it perceives you want to do.

You've heard the expression about computers, "garbage in, garbage out." The garbage that's going into the "things I want to happen" file in your mind contains all the nasty things you say about yourself (or what you hear others say about you that you don't reject as untrue). The "garbage out" is the result of your mind processing all the "in garbage" it receives and perceives as a directive. While "I must be getting old" might be a fleeting thought, your mind hears an emphasis on the word "must" and takes it as an order that getting old is something you want to do and must do.

It's just as damaging to say "I'm having a senior moment" as it is to say "I must be getting old"; "having" implies ownership. "I'm having a senior moment" is often said in such a prideful, self-deprecating way that it's akin to boasting that you enjoy and own it. The price of boasting about having a senior moment or trying to be charming is costly. If you tell yourself often enough that you are having a senior moment, it becomes an acceptable, embedded part of your thinking and affects how you function and how you age.

The word *senior* is a loaded bomb. In whatever sense you apply it to yourself, understand its power. Your mind takes in everything from the culture that relates to the word and uses it to shape and influence your thinking and behavior. *The less often you refer to yourself as a senior and the more often you reject the word as applying in any way to you, the more control you exert over your aging process.*

Another thing: if you mindlessly keep saying "I'm having a senior moment," you can expect to have more frequent memory lapses. These result not from an inability to recall but from fear and panic set off by unchecked repeated thinking or stating "I'm having a senior moment." It produces a kind of stress-induced brain freeze that public speakers experience when they lack confidence before an audience.

The whole "I'm having a senior moment" thing came about as a cutsie way to cover up suspected memory loss.

When I coach women about staying away from the "senior moment" language, they sometimes snap back, "Well, if my memory is failing, there is nothing I can do about it." They're wrong in thinking that nothing can be done about it. Part of the evil of "I'm having a senior moment" is that it implies that you are helpless against the loss of memory. You're not. There are so many mental and physical exercises that you can do to stay sharp.

You can do crossword puzzles or play mind games that are on the market. One of the best mind games is the Brain Fitness Program from Posit Science Corporation (see www.positscience.com) that has been featured on PBS. I have the program, use it, and love it. As sharp as I think I am, I have discovered that there is room for improvement, and measurable improvement does occur if you work with the program consistently. It should be standard software in every retirement community and senior center that has a computer.

There are also physically strengthening exercises that incorporate wonderful mental exercises; for example, tai chi requires you to learn increasingly complex forms. I recently signed up for a class to learn line dancing and found to my surprise that it takes more mental than physical effort. You really have to focus on what you're doing. Multitasker that I am, I discovered I can't write articles in my head while trying to learn dance steps!

One of the best things you can do to preserve or improve cognition is to fortify your nutrition with appropriate antioxidant supplements. If you take them well before suspected memory decline begins, they can go a long way toward prolonging mental competence. Even a cursory Internet investigation of the role of antioxidants in the prevention of Alzheimer's and other forms of cognitive decline turns up a long list of credible evidence indicating that specific supplements have prevention potential. Unfortunately, the medical establishment and pharmaceutical industry usually dismisses convincing research that shows the value of specific supplements.

I have never had a senior moment, and I never will. Why? Because I choose not to. Yes, I forget things and so does everyone else, young or not so young. I choose not to hammer my self-confidence over it.

When you feel the urge to declare "I'm having a senior moment," immediately correct yourself with "I know the answer. I'll give myself a moment—it will come to me." If the answer isn't forthcoming and you can't remember it, so what? It's less harmful than telling yourself over and over again that you're losing your mental competence and succumbing to decline.

Never Say "I'm Too Old"—You're Not Too Old!

It's bad enough if you use language of decline, but it's just as destructive if someone playfully tells you that you're getting old—and you do not immediately rebuke the statement as untrue. Your mind doesn't differentiate where the words it hears come from. If you allow your mind to be bombarded with too many "I'm too old" messages, you're going to start acting old whether you're forty-five or seventy-five.

Now you may deny that the "I'm too old" routine influences how you live, but you can probably relate countless ways that it's entered into decisions you've made. Be honest—has the thought "It's too late for me" *never* influenced a decision about doing something you wanted to do that traditionally isn't done at your age? Or, have you thought that you shouldn't do something because friends your age don't do it and they might scoff at you?

Instead of saying "I'm too old to do that," say "I can do anything," and watch what happens. It will light up your eyes and put a smile on your lips, and you will realize that you *can* do anything you choose to do. Chronological age be damned!

It's not pie in the sky. You *can* do what you *really* want to do. For example, perhaps you're close to retirement age but want to go back to school and become a doctor. A doctor, you say? Why not? If you're fifty and spend another ten years studying, you'll be sixty when you complete your degree. The best part is, if you're living a healthy, antiaging lifestyle, you'll have at least another twenty-five years to fulfill your dream and be of service to others. In the process, you'll enjoy the excitement, challenge, and benefit of being with young people.

Let's say you're forty-five, fifty-five, or even older and want to start your own business. Doing that may not be for everyone, but if you still have a fire in your belly, *go for it*. Ten years from now you could be the youthful CEO of a profitable business or a bored, mentally compromised retiree spending your days at the senior center reminiscing about what might have been. If you miss or reject an opportunity you may have now because of your age, I assure you that when you're in your late seventies or eighties and feeling fine, you will look back with regret. You will belatedly understand that at a healthy age of forty-five or fifty-five, you're still in the prime of your life.

It comes down to this: you have to reject all the "in garbage," regardless of its source. No matter how old you are chronologically, let your mind know clearly that you are not over the hill mentally or physically and have no desire to go there.

You are not "too old," so don't entertain thoughts that you "might" be too old! Live each day as if you believe you will live forever. Visualizing and living a "forever future" instead of "I'll be dead in X years so why should I have goals and dreams for the future" will make a huge difference in how much you enjoy life.

The next time you have to make a decision where age could be a factor, don't allow thoughts of "I'm too old" to affect the outcome. If you need some inspiration, consider these gutsy older entrepreneurs: Bob Axis, fifty-two, started

Certa Pro Painters in 2005; Silas Lumpkins, seventy-three, started Lumpkins Courier Service in 2004; Judy Finch, fifty-eight, started Echo Valley Campground in 1998; David White, fifty-three, started Heaven's Best Carpet and Upholstery Cleaning in 2001; Tom and Sue Ann McGoldrick, fifty-five and fifty-six, started Paws in Heaven Pet Funeral Home and Crematory.

You are what you say you are. You become what you say you are when you say it often enough. Refuse to talk yourself into decline. Using words that hasten deterioration is nothing to joke about. Using powerful, can-do thoughts, words, and actions supports your ability to manage your aging process.

About Alzheimer's

You may argue that all of this talk about controlling your thinking and self-talk is fine, but what happens if you develop Alzheimer's disease or another type of dementia? Even though you may be only in your forties or fifties, Alzheimer's is now prevalent enough that many people worry about it. If you've ever had to watch someone suffer from Alzheimer's or even the "normal" cognitive decline many older people experience, you might be thinking that nothing can be done.

Along with many nutrition-oriented physicians and researchers, I believe that we can avoid much of the usual cognitive decline *and* prevent Alzheimer's. My files are filled with credible evidence that indicates Alzheimer's can be prevented with adequate nutrition and specific antioxidant and other supplements, provided such intervention starts early enough. If this is a concern, educate yourself. Don't expect your physician to tell you everything you need to know. Chances are the only thing he or she will suggest is Aricept or another drug that is of limited value. (More about Aricept below.) I've already suggested an Internet investigation that will quickly turn up a variety of resources that should satisfy the most critical thinker.

In fighting or preventing cognitive decline, when is action "early enough"? Certainly, you take action when you become aware you don't remember things as well as you used to—not just once in a while, but often enough that it concerns you and others. For example, if you find yourself constantly dealing with forgetting where you put your keys, seek the help of a nutrition-oriented physician. He or she may be able to halt impending decline with adequate and specific supplements, improved diet and other interventions such as hormone adjustment. At the time of this writing, traditionally trained physicians can't prescribe drugs because none are available to stop early cognitive decline. Nor can traditionally trained physicians prescribe conventional drugs once dementia is established. In the resources section at the end of this book, you will find links that offer evidence that Alzheimer's may be preventable with specific supplements and antioxidant nutrition.

Unfortunately, inadequate funding prevents the pursuit of extensive nutrition-based research. When research indicates that something natural may work but needs additional study, the project usually dies. Most funding for non-drug research comes from the federal government and private foundations—and it's never enough. *What's more, organizations that advocate support for debilitating diseases generally don't adopt or defend natural approaches to prevention and cure.* They raise money for research and awareness purposes but rarely support nontraditional nutrition-oriented research. Their thinking seems to reflect a belief that what you do or do not put into your body doesn't matter all that much and cannot or does not impact a disease process. It's another example of "garbage in, garbage out," and I believe that this kind of thinking has some rather insidious roots. Getting old is big business. Debilitated old age is even bigger business.

Of course, the pharmaceutical industry participates in this "no cure" paradigm. It doesn't provide research funds for natural approaches to preventing Alzheimer's. What would they gain financially if they discovered an over-the-counter combination of supplements that could effectively prevent this disease? If the cure can't be patented, then the company can't turn a profit.

To date, there is absolutely no drug on the market that delays the onset of Alzheimer's or cures or stops the progression of the disease. Yes, advertising for a drug called Aricept claims to slow the progression of Alzheimer's, but many doctors disagree that it does. (See "Alzheimer's Drugs Which Work?" at www.medicinenet.com/script/main/art.

asp?articlekey=34241. Also see "Mild Cognitive Impairment May Signal Alzheimer's; Antioxidants Might Help Prevent It" at http://healthlink.mcw.edu/article/1031002487.html). I consider it misleading that Aricept is now advertised as being helpful in all stages of Alzheimer's. (Originally, it was promoted as helpful to delay the progression of the disease only in the early stage.) I have seen families without adequate insurance struggle to pay full retail price for Aricept under the mistaken belief and hope that the drug would help a failing parent avoid the inevitable. Had the parent lived an antiaging lifestyle, complete with a good diet, lots of physical and mental exercise, and appropriate supplements, the disaster may have been averted.

The infirmities that traditionally accompany old age are not foregone conclusions. You may not be able to prevent all health problems, but as long as you are mentally competent, you are in charge of what goes on in your head and how you live your life. You can help delay deterioration by avoiding decline-oriented language.

Choose Friends Carefully

Your Mother Was Right: Who You Hang With Matters!

O ne of the best ways to avoid adopting an old mind-set is to choose friends carefully. If you're fifty and associate with old-minded fifty-somethings, you'll be like them before you know it. Remember, you learn from each other. You copy each other's behaviors and adopt each other's thinking without even realizing it—for better or worse.

The effect of close association cannot be overlooked. A recent study on ABC News showed that if your friends are obese, you are likely to be obese as well ("Study: Obese Friends Could Make You Fat," July 25, 2007). On the other hand, if you choose to associate with people who value their lives and their bodies, you will likely do the same. Indeed, your mother was right when she shook her finger at you and admonished you not to associate with the bad neighborhood kids.

Not only do we become what we say we are, we become like those we associate with most often.

Even if you are the gutsiest, hippest, most non-conforming, fifty-plus role model in your group of old-oriented peers, social-straightjacket thinking will catch up with you. It will happen because ultimately it's easier to fit in than to buck the group mentality.

To stay young mentally, associate with younger people as well as those your age. This holds true whether you're in your forties, fifties, sixties, seventies, and beyond.

But here's the thing: you can't wait for young people to come to you. They prefer to associate with other young people, which is understandable because few have the maturity to value and nurture friendships with people older and presumably wiser than them. But there is a way around the dilemma, and you don't have to go clubbing to do it. You make a point to meet the younger people in your church, for instance. If you don't go to church, no problem. You can go back to school or volunteer to mentor young people. There is no shortage of ways to associate with those younger than you.

Most importantly, make a point to get to know the young people you work with. Don't look at them as competition for your job. That's old thinking, anyway. View young people as amazing sources of information and energy. I suggest you cannibalize their energy—feed on it because it's free and just what you need to stimulate your youthful energy juices!

More than the benefits of the energy young people exude, I know from personal experience the value of what you can relearn from them. They can be extraordinary teachers. In the workplace they are patient, tolerant, and understanding. They will bend over backwards to help. On more than one occasion at the pharmacy, I have relied on younger staff members to defuse a situation brewing with an obnoxious, demanding customer. I simply asked one of the young technicians to take over. They listen, empathize, and take a lot of guff that I wouldn't—without thinking anything of it. It's all in a day's work to them. Their attitude and behavior constantly remind me to be more patient and understanding, especially when challenged by difficult people.

This is so important that I'll say it one more time: *If you want to maintain a young attitude and outlook on life, be with youthful people.* You won't always like what you see or hear; you may be dismayed by some of their ideas and behaviors. But you will benefit from their energy, enthusiasm, and openness. Your interactions with them will likely turn on the light in your eyes and fill you with more youthful energy. It will force you to reassess the stodgy, straightjacket thinking that society foists on you as you progress through the stages of aging.

If you happen to be single, you'll also find a bonus to this strategy: if you maintain a young outlook while seeking a significant other, your chances of catching a "live one" escalate astronomically!

Strategy No. 6:
Beware of the
Senior Culture Club

Just Say "No" to Anything "Senior"

A ll of my advice up to this point and throughout the rest of the book comes down to this one strategy. It is the pivotal point around which you either successfully live an antiaging lifestyle or not.

In most countries, the senior culture is hard to ignore or escape. Made up of a powerful brotherhood/sisterhood in which only the old gain entry, it welcomes you with open arms once you reach fifty years of age or younger. You know you are nearing eligibility when you receive your first invitation to join AARP.

It's tempting to become part of the senior culture because it offers so many enticing activities and special perks (for example, seniors' discounts, access to government/ community services and programs, seniors-only housing, seniors-only publications). The seniors-only designation also gives the impression that you belong to an exclusive club, and many older people are drawn to that. However, sometimes that exclusiveness breeds an "us against the world" attitude, and that sense of exclusivity breeds ever-increasing amounts of acceptance—that is, acceptance of being old.

If you're in your forties, you might be thinking, "What are you talking about? What senior culture? I'm nowhere near the age where I would live in a senior community or go to a senior center for my entertainment." But be aware that even at age forty you're beginning to receive subtle messages from all over the place, luring you ever closer into the trap of seniorhood. The senior culture is a place where everybody seems to go sooner or later. The good news is that *you* don't have to join them!

How and Why It Ages You

Just as you must constantly be aware of other aging behaviors, you must always be on the lookout for the messages that the Senior Culture Club is sending you. It can be seductive, but know this: the senior culture is a vehicle for decline. In the senior culture, you interact primarily with others your own age, with similar mind-sets and circumstances. You learn from each other, unconsciously copying behaviors, beliefs, and attitudes. You bond with each other and support each other. You adopt consensus senior thinking. You buy into the socially accepted and heavily promoted senior lifestyle and mind-set. What are you really doing? *You are learning how to get old with each other in an exclusive club that breeds oldness and decline.*

What a terrible thing to say! How can the senior culture be a negative influence on the aging process? Aren't there stimulating, youthful activities within the senior culture that promote personal growth and good health? Absolutely. For example, organizations such as Oasis offer a wide variety of excellent programs that benefit seniors; it would be foolish not to use them. Then what is the problem?

The problem is not with individual programs, organizations, or activities. It's not just the separatist mind-set and lifestyle. It's all the parts of the senior culture, taken as a whole, that promote traditional, group-oriented attitudes, beliefs, and behaviors. *When the collective power of this club becomes a dominant influence in an older person's life, he or she will age traditionally.*

This is why I'm cautioning you about this now. In order to live agelessly, you must have unrestricted openness to the world and an independent spirit that resists conformity and consensus thinking. Ageless aging requires you to *live seamlessly, in a constant state of growth and productivity* (even if "retired"), all the while ignoring your chronological age. Growth occurs when an activity has a defined purpose, is productive, and has a goal. The contemporary senior culture cannot support or promote growth because, by its very nature, it is decline oriented. If you doubt that seamless growth is vital, remember that what doesn't grow, quickly deteriorates and dies.

The senior culture has become what it is primarily because of a long-established cultural understanding that age sixty-five and beyond is a period of decline. This belief is based on an antiquated and erroneous assumption that ability and desire to grow and produce cease with advancing age. Considering how some (if not many) people age, it makes a modicum of sense. However, it also denies the reality that many sixty-five-year-olds are mentally and physically competent and will stay that way for a long period of time. They should be encouraged and helped to realize their full potential, instead of wasting it in traditional retirement.

More than any other reason, the senior culture is what it is because of the misguided government policy established during the Great Depression that determined sixty-five as the appropriate age to retire. It may have made sense when sixty-five was about as long as people lived, but today it makes no sense at all.

I know that traditional retirement will always be a part of our culture, and it should be because not everyone can or wants to work forever. We are all different and have different desires and abilities. Nevertheless, traditional retirement has become an anachronism and a financial albatross.

Why an anachronism? As I previously mentioned, in the past century the life span has increased by thirty years. In 1900, the life expectancy was 47.3 years. According to the Centers for Disease Control and Prevention (CDC), in 2002 that number had risen to 77.3 years. In the face of this truth, people still begin traditional retirement at age sixty-five and earlier. Those folks will have a lot of extra years in which to do something or nothing with their lives. How will they spend those bonus years? Will they have enough money? Not likely, judging by the number of retirees who struggle to make ends meet very early in retirement. (See "Making Ends Meet," *U.S. News & World Report*, June 2008.)

Traditional retirement is becoming a financial albatross for a couple of reasons. First, we've been warned that Social Security will be bankrupt in the near future. Second, the baby boomer generation is beginning to retire. Are all boomers prepared financially? Not likely. Many boomers grudgingly say that they plan to work past retirement age because they can't afford to retire. They may not understand that if they are healthy, this is the best action they could take. Not only will they stay healthier longer and have a better quality of life, but they will also avoid being sucked too deeply into the decline-oriented senior culture.

I would caution boomers: it's not enough to intend to work; you need to know what you will work at. The same boring stuff you've done all your life? Any old job that provides a paycheck? Or, something you've always wanted to do but couldn't because you were busy earning a living? Those boomers who plan to work should have a postretirement plan. This is not just a financial plan, but a plan for living productively—not just existing.

Insurance ads tell working people that they need a financial plan for retirement so they know where they're going. That message is good but incomplete. So what if you have a great financial plan for retirement. How will you spend your time and money? On cruises, golfing, or living life as a pastime in a seniors-only community with other people of the same age and circumstances? How depressing! No, it's worse than depressing—it's deadly. When you don't grow and produce, you deteriorate sooner than you need to.

We Need an Alternative Culture

In addition to traditional retirement, we need to establish a parallel or alternative culture that legitimizes and supports those folks at retirement age whose early planning has resulted in a productive, balanced, postretirement second life. Creating this culture will require a huge cultural shift and a new social mind-set, but it has to happen. We can't afford to lose so much valuable elder potential to rocking chairs and golf courses.

Many people spend their working lives in jobs they hate or find unfulfilling, and at retirement they lament that they wish they could have done something else all those years. At retirement you can always decide to do what you've always wanted, but age sixty-five is not the time to plan how you want to spend the rest of your life. You are tired, and the carefree senior culture is inviting you to join. It's too easy to cave in and vegetate with your peers who are living life as a pastime.

At age forty, insurance agents and financial planners are available to sell you a policy or give investment advice for retirement, but there is no one to help you plan for the life you've always wanted. We know that sixty-five is no longer "old." For many people, sixty-five could be the beginning of the most rewarding part of their lives, if only they had planned for it or had the help to do so.

Insurance companies and independent financial planners are missing the boat. They are missing out financially by not helping clients create a productive, postretirement life plan. In addition to selling financial plans, they can sell "life after work" productivity plans. We have coaches for every imaginable need. Life coaches, work coaches, team coaches, travel coaches. Why not life-after-work coaches? We have plenty of successful older people who can lead the way in how to do it. By tapping into their expertise, we can help preretirees achieve their postretirement goals.

To be a bit facetious, perhaps our approach to aging as well as the senior culture itself is a good thing for the economy. As I have pointed out already, aging is big business, especially debilitated old age. There is probably more profit in dealing with decline than in promoting and supporting growth. If people were encouraged to stay productive as long as they could or wanted to, many businesses that provide supportive retirement and senior services would disappear. What I question now, however, is what has disappeared because the Senior Culture Club is nowadays so clearly defined.

When I was growing up, there was no such thing as a senior culture or anything even remotely similar to what we have now. Today, many old and even not-so-old people live in whisper-quiet, walled-in, gated communities in tiny "villas" surrounded only by clones of themselves. Sights or sounds of youth are evident only when grandkids come to visit or when a feisty resident geezer roars his Harley past the villas, hoping to attract the attention of lonely resident widows. Although these enclaves are usually esthetically attractive, the sight of perfectly manicured lawns and expansive vistas often eerily resembles a memorial park.

In times past, old people remained in the diverse community they lived in all their lives, usually as part of an extended family or near caring relatives or neighbors. The closest thing to a retirement community was the "old folk's home" where indigents lived out their last days. There were no senior centers for old people to segregate themselves and feed off each other's oldness. There were no senior publications featuring ads for cemeteries, wills, dentures, and diapers—all reminders that the end is near. *The elderly were not yet big business.*

Instead of seeking companionship in a senior center, old people were viable parts of the community. For entertainment and connection with others, they often sat on the front porches of their homes, where they interacted with families and young people in the community. The old shared their wisdom, and the young provided energy and excitement; everyone benefited. It could be argued that the culture of the time didn't offer opportunities for growth that exist today for older people, and unfortunately, that's true. However, at least the elderly were not separated from the rest of the world, which was teeming with energizing life. They maintained their unique personalities, behaviors, and beliefs rather than conforming to a stagnating and controlling group mentality.

I know that my take on the senior culture may sound harsh, and many might take offense at it. However, no offense is intended. Those in the senior culture who are living happy, satisfying, traditional senior lifestyles are entitled to live how they choose, without criticism.

However, since I wrote this book for women in their forties and fifties who want to stay ageless indefinitely, you are not and hopefully never will be "seniors." Furthermore, most of you aren't even close to being old mentally or physically, but you need to grab hold of the reality of what's ahead. Know that you have a choice about how you can live in your older years—if you prepare now. If only we could *really* grasp the power of choice that we can exert!

Why I Won't Join the Club

Because I am so adamant about this point, let me give you some perspective on how and why I perceive the senior culture as I do. I am not now nor have I ever been a member of the Senior Culture Club. I never had the desire or time to join. So how can I pass judgment on something I've never been a part of? The answer is that during my years working as a pharmacist, I saw many aspects of the senior culture, often in intimate detail. I didn't have to experience it to understand it. Observation is a great teacher if you pay attention to what you see and hear.

The last pharmacy I worked in had a large senior clientele. I was as old or older than most of the customers, yet I couldn't identify with them. When I interacted with them, I felt like an outsider looking in on a depressing culture, and I was unable to empathize with how they were living. It was a strange feeling.

Most of the people were in a traditional retired lifestyle, which was apparent in their thinking, appearance, and demeanor. I got to know most of them well enough to evaluate what their lives were like, and as a result I was thankful each day that I was still working. As I've already mentioned, I always gratefully thought, "There but for the grace of God go I." Never did I envy their seemingly carefree lifestyle; there was nothing about it that I found appealing. Experiencing the reality of so much decline on a daily basis motivated me to stay productive and to keep up my antiaging lifestyle.

For example, while my coworkers were compromising their health by feasting on chips, soda, and cookies during the day, I usually dined on raw cashews (my favorite) and drank plenty of water. There was never enough time to sit down for a decent meal, anyway. When I got home from work, even if I was dog tired, I immediately walked on the treadmill for thirty minutes and lifted some weights. It restored my energy and got the blood moving out of my legs, which I had been on for ten to twelve hours.

Remember earlier when I told you that women younger than me would lament, "Barbara, don't ever get old"? I understood what they meant. Their lives were pleasant for the most part, but they were definitely in decline. I used to wonder how their lives might be different if they were still productive, working, or engaged in activities that mentally and physically challenged them and kept them growing.

A few of the older women (and fewer men) were still working. Most of the retired women were content that they were at home. A common remark was, "I've worked hard all my life, and I deserve my retirement." Everybody deserves their retirement, but the human mind and body are not designed to lie fallow. Either you use it or you lose it. It's a cliché, but it's painfully true.

More important, the difference between the employed and the retirees was significant. The workers were in better condition physically and they were mentally sharper. They dealt with their health problems as just another bump in the road—not something to dwell on excessively—as many old people with little else to occupy their time often do. The workers radiated a level of energy not normally seen at their age; their speech came easily, and they moved with confidence. Their appearance was contemporary. Their lifestyle would not be for everyone, but it was clear that more than a few of the retired women would rather have been out in the world with them.

In fact, a few women who were ready to give up the boredom of retirement told me that they wished they had a job but thought, "At my age, what could I do?" The obvious answer is *plenty*. You can always go back to school to learn marketable skills. I often made that suggestion, but in most cases it wasn't well received. Responses tended to be in the nature of "It's too late for me." It's never too late if you are mentally and physically competent, but for some, a lack of self-confidence can be an insurmountable roadblock.

Entertainment in the Senior Culture Club feeds into that lack of self-confidence and inability to self-start. I despise much of senior entertainment for one reason: so much of it focuses on living life as a pastime. Cruises for those who can afford them, golf for those still agile enough to swing a club, shopping, doctor visits, and socializing at senior centers. In California, casino-sponsored buses pick up seniors at retirement centers and designated areas around town to take them out for a day of gambling and eating. I have nothing against gambling for those with money to waste, but picking the pockets of seniors on fixed incomes and calling it entertainment is unacceptable. I recall one situation at the pharmacy when a woman on welfare objected to a small co-pay for her medication because she said she needed the money to gamble.

For several reasons, many seniors are not self-starters; they rely on others to direct and select activities. For example, my local Oasis program offers exercise classes for seniors. Old bodies need exercise as much or more than young bodies, but these classes are not well attended. Why? Because no one has organized and provided transportation to the classes. The casinos would perform a valuable service if in addition to transporting seniors to gamble, they would also take seniors to Oasis classes and other programs that would improve quality of life.

Regardless of age, people are happier when they're productive and feel they have a reason for their existence. They are even happier when they're mentally competent, financially secure, and in charge of their lives. Living life as a pastime does not promote that state of being.

How to Avoid the Senior Culture

Even though your "retirement" might be years away, you are either close to or are at the age when you're starting to get invitations to join the senior culture. Remember, the invitations and cultural messages are very seductive. You need to decide now that you will not be one of those retirees who wishes she was still out there in the world mixing it up with all kinds of people and enjoying energizing challenges.

To overcome the lure of the senior culture, first accept that it exists and then deliberately avoid plugging into it. When you reach "senior" age, don't stick your head in the sand and pretend it doesn't exist. Use what it offers to advance your growth and productivity (for example, computer and investment classes are useful). However, while doing so, stay firm in your intention that you will not become part of the senior culture or establish an emotional connection or identity with it.

If you unintentionally move into the Senior Culture Club and don't like it, don't wait too long to choose a different lifestyle; the longer you stay, the more difficult it is to leave. The club offers a level of comfort, camaraderie, and security that is appealing to the older mind and body.

Most important, consciously work to lessen the influence of the senior culture on your life. Start by shifting your ideas about how you perceive advanced age, a process that requires you to change in the following ways:

- You reject identification or classification as a senior. Instead, you always see and portray yourself as ageless. You keep in the forefront of your consciousness the ageless person you want to be and the life you want to live.

- You avoid as much as possible seniors-only communities, as well as seniors-only activities, organizations, and publications. The seniors-only communities make sense only when you need an assisted living arrangement because you're no longer able to care for yourself—and that will hopefully be many, many years down the road (if ever).

- You build friendships with and engage in activities with younger people.

- You resolve to stay productive as long as possible. Living on Social Security is akin to living in poverty. A fixed income that forces you to count every penny creates a deprived, dependent spirit and a lifestyle that is aging.

How do you derail an unintended slide into the senior culture and the deterioration it aids and abets? *Be the boss of what goes on in your head.*

- Every day, stay oriented to the future, not the past. (It's gone, so don't live in it.)

- Set exciting goals that force you to grow, learn, and *produce,* regardless of your age, even if you choose to retire from the workforce. Adopt role models, and look for mentors to motivate you and keep you focused on reaching your goals.

- Choose to be an innovative leader, not a follower of trends and outdated traditions.

Think and Prepare Now

In summary, no one can or wants to work forever. At some point you must find a balance between work and having a life. Well before your chosen time of retirement, you can decide to define the meaning of that period of time that's right for you. You can decide that it will mean that you stop doing what you've done all of your life (and perhaps hated) and instead, begin to live a rich, exciting, fulfilling, productive second life. To accomplish this takes a lot of preplanning, which is why I encourage you to take a hard look at it now when you can do so much to ensure an ageless future for yourself. If you can find a life-after-work coach to help you, so much the better. If not, you can do it on your own. (See http://plus50connect.com/resources.htm.)

Where do you start? I recommend two books for all future-oriented preretirees to read. The first is *Don't Stop the Career Clock* by Helen Harkness, PhD. The other is *Bold Retirement: Mining Your Own Silver for a Rich Life* by Mary Lloyd. These titles are more than books; they are how-to road maps to help you plan the future you desire. They are unique in that they provide tools to help you figure out what you really want to do with the rest of your life. They are also written with a profound clarity, common sense, and degree of guidance that you have undoubtedly never before encountered. So many books are touted as "life changing." These two books truly have that potential if you are serious about creating the life you want in your postretirement years. And by the way, if you're already into retirement and want to change the direction of your life, it's not too late to benefit from these books. They are lifesavers for floundering retirees.

The "Used to Be Trap"

Before I end this chapter, I want you to be aware of one more nasty trap that the Senior Culture Club sets for you; moreover, I want you to internalize a barrier to it. It is *vital* to understand that after you retire from your present work, you can't allow yourself to become or think of yourself as a "used to be" or "has-been." This is true even if people ask, "Didn't you used to be a teacher?" or "Didn't you used to be a lawyer?" or "Didn't you used to be a nurse?" Those are the kinds of questions that get asked in Senior Culture Club gatherings.

The "didn't you used to be" question can be painful to hear and can seriously decimate your self-worth—unless you realize that all the "used to be" people are still who they were before they retired. And if you plan wisely you can say, "I still am the person I used to be, but I've also become the person I've always wanted to be. Now I have the life that I've always wanted. And by the way, how can I help you with what I know?"

Whatever your age, don't ever allow awareness of passing years and the winding down of life to plunge you into depression or sadness about what might have been. If you plan properly, that won't happen. Turn your awareness of where you are in life right now into determination to live life fully. Do it starting *now*. Prepare legally for the inevitable, and then live each day as if you believe you will live forever. Visualizing and acting on a "forever future" instead of "I'll be dead in X years so why should I have long-range goals or dreams for the future" will make a huge difference in how much you enjoy life. I cannot stress this concept too much—it's so potent and powerful when you internalize it and live by it.

If at any time you despair about being able to have the kind of future you really want, consider the following ageless icons who are living the lives they want because they prepared well and knew what they had to do to stay in the game. I reveal their ages because they are well known, and I want to encourage you not to be concerned about your chronological age. I'll bet that if the ages of the following people were not known, they wouldn't ask anyone to guess how old they are. Only Little Old Ladies and Little Old Geezers do that.

- Art Linkletter: At ninety-plus he is actively involved in multiple business projects and has a full speaking schedule. With Mark Victor Hansen he recently coauthored *How to Make the Rest of Your Life the Best of Your Life*. I am pleased to share that I was interviewed for their book and am quoted often throughout its pages.

- Tony Bennett: seventy-plus and still going strong. The twinkle in his eyes while he sings tells it all: he's living his passion and that's a lesson for all us. When you are living your best life, it turns on the light in your eyes and fills your soul with joy.

- David Oreck: A remarkable eighty-plus role model, Oreck is active in his company doing commercials for his vacuum cleaners. He's an example of what men at his age can be when they remain productive.

- Helen Harkness: An ageless woman who never reveals her age, Harkness conducts her own business, Career Design Associates in Garland, Texas. I have had the privilege of meeting Dr. Harkness, and she has become a motivating force in my life. Not only does she actively operate her own business, she also speaks, writes, and travels all over the world. At her age, many traditional women are in retirement homes, having left life behind in unfulfilled dreams. She is the author of *Don't Stop the Career Clock* and other valuable books.

- Mary Lloyd: In her vibrant sixties, Mary is the author of *Bold Retirement: Mining Your Own Silver for a Rich Life*. A woman of uncommon wisdom and experience, she has a way of thinking and looking at life that is uniquely thought provoking. But more than that, she shares resources in her book that everyone needs to profitably navigate the older years—tools that few people have access to.

- Regis Philbin: At seventy-five, he is easily taken for much younger, if for no other reason than he works at being contemporary and soaks up the energy of his thirty-something cohost. While talking to and interacting with young celebrities (which would be boring to most people his age), Reeg does what he does—and obviously loves to do—to stay in the game. As I watch him, I am amazed at his quick wit as he parries with guests and off-camera people. There is nothing "old" about him.

* * *

If you are a youthful, healthy person aged forty to fifty, you *can* stay at that level of wellness and youthfulness for at least another twenty-five years—and even *improve* your health during that time. You can get to sixty-five, seventy-five, and beyond with the same strength, stamina, and vitality you have now. The above-mentioned ageless icons have done that.

Many unforeseen events will influence, shape, and even detour your ageless journey. But in spite of these setbacks and roadblocks, you will be far, far ahead of your peers if you can maintain a detachment from the trappings and enticements of the Senior Culture Club and live the kind of future you really want.

You can decide how you want to live and
be now and in the future when you have
a plan and make informed choices.

Strategy No. 7:
Protect Your Youth from Culture Vultures

Don't Play the Numbers Game

Now that you're more fully aware of the Senior Culture Club, we need to look more closely at how we have been trained to act—culturally—around old people and even not-so-old people.

I can understand that you might be proud of how you look, that you feel that you look so good for your age that you want everyone to know. However, as you age, understand this: every time you verbalize your age, you reinforce the social significance (and your own awareness) of your chronological age. That means you shouldn't tell your age if you care about how people respond to you or think about you.

There is a huge difference between others *guessing* your exact age and others *knowing* your exact age. The minute you tell your age, you expose yourself to the biases, perceptions, and expectations others have about how you ought to be. The result? They treat you accordingly, which you may not like. Everyone, and I do mean everyone, has a stereotypical image of what people should look like, act like, think like, dress like, and be like at a given age.

Knowing the actual age of a person always plays into your interactions with them.

Your age is nobody's business. But people are curious. When they get to know you, they really want to know your age, even if they say it doesn't matter. Beware: it *does* matter. Knowing your age gives people a sense of how they could or should deal with you. Despite others' best intentions, it's difficult to treat you without regard for your age because those darned stereotypical biases that everyone has that affect how we deal with one another.

Bottom line: to the extent possible, keep your age to yourself. You want others to interact with you as the ageless person you are and project yourself to be—not based on the number of years you have lived.

In the workplace, age can matter a lot. Why? Because we live in an ageist society. This means that as a culture we are prejudiced against age. While it's unacceptable to discriminate because of race, gender, or sexual preference, discrimination because of age happens all the time.

The government can pass every antidiscrimination law possible, but in many business situations, knowledge of your age can change the outcome of a promotion if age forty or beyond is considered "old" in those environments. If a woman looks younger and can keep her age to herself (admittedly very difficult to do!), she holds a winning hand. It's too bad it's this way; it just shows that all the blather about equal rights means nothing because age can and too often does become a deal breaker.

The main problem with age discrimination is that it is often couched in the belief that "I was just helping." To illustrate, let me share a story. An older pharmacist friend was working in a pharmacy where her age was not an issue because it wasn't known. Her fellow pharmacists and technicians, mostly young, accepted her without question or qualification. She was one of the team. Then one day, an article about her volunteer work appeared in the local newspaper, and it, unfortunately, revealed her age. Almost immediately, her age became a topic of conversation at work. Her coworkers couldn't believe that she was "that" old.

Her supervisor called to tell her that he'd seen the story and that he had "no idea" she was as old as she was (in a tone that suggested she had a terminal disease). He asked, "Lucy, when do you intend to retire?" She replied, "Never." They both laughed, but that wasn't the end of it. Every time they spoke after that conversation, he asked when she planned to retire. Every time she gave the same answer: "never." It became a running joke.

Several months later, the pharmacy manager resigned and Lucy assumed that she'd be offered the position because she had seniority. Her supervisor called and said, "Lucy, as you know, Mark is leaving. You're an outstanding pharmacist—a superstar—and we're lucky to have you." (Elated, Lucy thought he was getting ready to offer the position.) "But Lucy, we don't want to overtax you (i.e., "You're too old" or "I just want to help you avoid being overworked"), so we're bringing in a pharmacist who wants to relocate to this area. She'll be the new pharmacy manager." The position went to a young, newly licensed pharmacist.

Should Lucy have fought this decision? No. It wouldn't have been worth the trouble. In addition to losing the battle, she would have created animosity and a hostile work environment. One of the blessings of maturity is realizing that life is short, so it's smart to pick battles carefully. But please don't lose the point of this story. In the workplace, awareness of your age does matter, *particularly* if you're an older woman trying to shatter that legendary glass ceiling.

Stop Ageism Now!

The only way to stop this kind of prejudicial thinking is to be vocal about it before it can happen. Just as we had to fight for our rights as women, we're going to have to band together and fight for our rights no matter what our age.

Here's a radical idea: in California, a law allows students and school staff to define their own perceived identity, appearance, or behavior. Taking that a step further, I think the time has come for individuals to have the right to legally define and live their perceived age. (It's a challenging proposition fraught all kinds of legal issues, but when there's a will, there's a way.) Why be bound by chronological age and the negative baggage attached to it when you feel and are able to function as you did when you were years younger?

If it were legal to live one's perceived age, if that were upheld as a cultural norm and a civil right, life would be vastly different in the workplace as well as in social situations. It would be a given that judgment about suitability for promotions and pay raises *must* be made based not on age but on performance and competence. This is not to be naïve and think that age prejudice would cease to exist. We live in an imperfect world with imperfect people. It may take an effort the magnitude of the civil rights movement to effect change, but it can be done.

Fortunately, the outlook for change is in our favor. I predict that because of the size of the aging population and the shortage of adequately trained, English-speaking young people needed for highly skilled positions, positive change in how a chronologically older person is treated in the workplace may happen sooner than expected. In many businesses, there is no substitute for experience. That we are making progress in this area, see the MetLife Foundation/ Civic Ventures Encore Career Survey at www.encore.org/ news/encore-career-survey-enc.

However, know that we're fighting a nasty battle with some powerful but seemingly innocuous enemies. We may win the right in court to legally say our perceived age, but it's the cultural forces that drive ageist thinking that are the most harmful and the most difficult to change. I touched on this in the section about the senior culture in Strategy No. 6, but I'm elaborating here because you need to be aware of what you must fight.

The significance of advancing age as a serious social, business, and personal issue begins to kick into high gear around age fifty. The "you are getting old" messages start in earnest at age forty, but by age fifty they really hit you hard. They come from everywhere—from TV ads to insurance companies, from so-called friends (the ones who send you "over the hill" reminders on your birthday), to even your own personal perceptions of yourself.

TV ads are probably the most egregious offenders, particularly those from drug companies. At age fifty or thereabouts, the drug companies start to portray you as a senior and point their advertising guns straight at your mind. They suggest that you need drugs to treat osteoporosis, insomnia, dry eyes, heartburn, constipation, arthritis, incontinence, restless legs, depression, and even Alzheimer's disease—all ailments typically suffered by old people. So, even if you're forty and have arthritis symptoms, for example, the ads clearly imply that you're old or getting old. Such ads can have a tremendous impact on how you think about yourself at this time of your life.

At age fifty, insurance company ads suggest that you're a senior who will soon enter traditional retirement. Advertisements show youngish, white-haired men and women, sweaters wrapped around their shoulders, playing golf, fishing, and generally living life as a pastime—as many old people still do. If you factor into such ads promotions for retirement communities for those "fifty or better," it's tough not to unwittingly adopt a senior mind-set and begin to think of yourself as growing old.

From personal experience, having been age fifty some twenty-nine years ago, I clearly recall what that was like. At age fifty you look back to the time you were thirty. You realize you're getting on. Not getting old—just getting on. Because you haven't yet experienced life in the future, you don't realize how young you still are. Furthermore, you won't appreciate that until you live another twenty years.

At age fifty you know without a doubt that inside you are still as young as you were twenty years ago, but the cultural messages suggest or directly state that you're getting old. That's what I experienced. The only thing different today is that at age fifty there are many more intense, pervasive, and subliminal "you are getting old" messages bombarding you daily. They seep into your mind as if by osmosis, and if you're not on guard they can negatively shape your perception of yourself and how you live.

Bottom line: if you're fifty or younger, stay alert for the constant assaults on your youth. Teach yourself to recognize and filter out "you are getting old" messages, whatever their source. Be on guard against ageist behavior, and most important, don't allow any of this to take root in your mind. Be aware once again that old age, particularly debilitated old age, is big business. The sooner the debilitated-old-age net can reel you in, the more lucrative it is for the senior culture vultures to grab your money and your youth.

When you're age forty or fifty and the old-age industry suggests or directly states that you are getting old, deliberately affirm the truth that you are not old. You are not old until you allow yourself to be.

Take a stand! No more culturally created Little Old Ladies!

Celebrate Birth Dates, Not Years Gone By

Birthday Parties Are for Kids

Okay, I admit it. I'm a radical at heart, but I want to pick up one of the points I just made and look at it in depth: the idea of being allowed to live your perceived age legally and culturally.

If you could live your perceived age—and no one kept track of the years that have gone by—how do you think you would be living? Stop and think about it. How would your life be different? How would *you* be different? Other than physical changes, you'd have few reminders that the end is near. You would be open to more opportunities to live life more fully. *You and your life would be liberated beyond measure.* Stop for a moment, and savor that idea. Really think about what it could mean to you.

For example, imagine that if you lived your perceived age you could free yourself from the tyranny of birthday celebrations. Birthday parties are for kids! After childhood, birthday parties serve only as reminders that you're rapidly approaching the final curtain.

So here's my idea. Stop celebrating the years that have gone by. Instead, celebrate your birth date—every month of the year—*by doing something to help you stay ageless.* Get out your appointment book, and write down the details of what you'll do on a specific day each month.

For example if your birth date is the twenty-seventh, then on the twenty-seventh of each month you might do the following:

January 27:	Drink at least eight eight-ounce glasses of water. Do it today and every day. It's fabulous for your skin. At home or work, keep a gallon bottle of water nearby and drink at least half of it every day. After it becomes a daily habit, you will look and feel younger.
February 27:	If you haven't yet cleaned up your diet by eliminating excessive amounts of processed stuff, don't wait another day—skip the fast food. One fewer meal at McDonald's every week won't kill you. In fact, it will help you control your weight.
March 27:	Sign up for a gym membership. Better yet, purchase a treadmill, put it in front of your TV, and use it every day without fail. Instead of sitting on the sofa and snacking while you watch your favorite TV programs, walk!

April 27:   You've been exercising and eating less junk, so you've lost weight. Now go buy some updated clothes that fit you well. Get a new hair color, and go for a young-looking hairstyle.

May 27:   Subscribe to a newsletter that will help you stay healthy. (See the resources section for suggestions.)

June 27:   Make an appointment with your dentist. If you haven't seen a dentist in a while and your teeth have fallen into disrepair, this should be the first thing on your list. Get them whitened if possible. Nothing says "old" more than yellow teeth.

July 27:   Sign up for a class that interests you at the local community college. You will meet and associate with young people, and you'll keep your brain sharp by learning something new.

August 27:   Take a minivacation at a spa to get rid of stress that's assaulting your mind and body. Or take a real vacation away from phones, TV, and the Internet.

September 27:   If you're unhappy with your appearance, especially your face, make an appointment with a cosmetic surgeon. Minor tweaking may be all you need to significantly improve your appearance. If the skin on your face has the appearance of cross-hatching, ask your doctor for a prescription for Retin-A. It can make the surface of your skin smooth as silk when you use it safely and properly. It won't do much for wrinkles, however.

October 27: If you haven't already done, so make an appointment with an antiaging physician. You can find one in your area at the website for the American College for Advancement of Medicine (see /www.ACAM.org).

November 27: Buy more clothes if you've lost more weight—or just because it's fun!

December 27: What the heck, it's Christmas. Have some eggnog! Commit to getting back on track January 2.

The previous activities are just suggestions. I want you to create your own agenda to celebrate the day of your birth, not that you are getting older. Celebrate that you are alive and living a vital, full life. Above all, make it a fun and future-oriented way to help stay ageless!

Strategy No. 9:
Adopt the New Stages of Aging

The Ultimate Key to Ageless Aging

When does "middle age" start? Fifty years ago it may have been appropriate to call anyone who reached age fifty or fifty-five "middle-aged" or even a "senior," but it no longer makes sense. As I've already mentioned, we're living longer—thirty years longer in the past century. However, it takes cultural perceptions quite a bit more time to catch up with statistics. In the process of thinking about this book, I asked a number of women in their fifties whether they thought of themselves as middle-aged. Interestingly, the majority of these women, especially the ones who had been consciously living a healthy lifestyle, emphatically said no to the question.

Unfortunately, we traditionally go through the aging process not trying to manage it to our advantage but just allowing life to happen. As a result, by the time most people reach what is traditionally called "middle age," they are resigned to simply let life take its course. They increasingly become more accepting of the fact that they are declining. By the time they get to their golden years, they're existing more than they're living. That could and should change.

But doing so will require a new take on how we look at stages of aging.

Fortunately, Dr. Helen Harkness has provided a workable guide in her groundbreaking book *Don't Stop the Career Clock*. In it she offers a new realistic and liberating way to live stages of aging that should be adopted—if not by society then certainly by individuals. Dr. Harkness writes, "If we need some kind of aging chronology, I suggest we design our own." Here's her "live long, die fast" contemporary model for categorizing the aging process:

- Young adulthood: 20–40
- First midlife: 40–60
- Second midlife: 60–80
- Young-old: 80–90
- Elderly: 90 and above
- Old-old: 2–3 years to live

Is this chronology realistic? Absolutely. Census figures show that in 1950, possibly 2,300 centenarians lived in the United States. Today, more than 40,000 centenarians make up our population. By 2050, close to a million people will be one hundred years of age or older. The Harkness chronology makes sense not just because people are living longer but also because many are living healthier lives. If it's become a cliché that "today's sixty is yesterday's forty"—which is true—then why do we put up with traditional thinking and behaviors about aging that are as archaic as the "earth is flat" theory?

Imagine this: if you are fifty and adopt the Harkness model, you don't have to think of yourself or behave as middle-aged. You are simply in your *first* midlife. If you are sixty-five, you aren't elderly (as society currently labels you); you're simply in your *second* midlife. Adopting the Harkness chronology makes a huge difference in how you see yourself, how you embrace your potential, and how you live your life. Why?

- It validates the youthful person you are inside, regardless of your *actual* age.

- It enables you to live your *perceived* age.

- It is truly liberating.

So I challenge you. The next time someone asks you the dreaded "how old are you" question, you answer with "I'm in my first midlife." They may look at you funny, but at least you have opened the door to having a conversation about it, which is key to changing a culture's mind-set. We make up our culture, and it is up to us—not some other powers that be—to decide whether what we say is culturally acceptable. Starting conversations about the way we view our life stages is a way to start getting people comfortable with changing their beliefs about what is "middle age" and what is "old."

Strategy No. 10:

Refuse to Age Gracefully

Only Old Broads and Little Old Ladies Do It

L et's assume that you develop a perpetual awareness of what you want to be like twenty-five years from now. You fully understand the pitfalls of an "I'm too old to do that" mentality. You now see your future self, whatever your actual age, in a new light. You adopt the Harkness model as a positive way to live and talk about where you are chronologically speaking. The next step in getting the right antiaging mind-set is getting the right attitude. Yes, it's a tired, old cliché, but it's true. *Attitude is everything.*

Let me be blunt. You have to *work hard* at keeping a youthful attitude. Why? Because everything in our society militates against it. I've warned you about the power of the decline-oriented senior culture and the importance of avoiding it. As you reach your traditional, middle-aged years, senior culture customs dictate that you think, act, dress, walk, and talk in socially accepted, senior ways. Even if you deliberately avoid opting into the senior culture, its mores are pervasive.

As I cautioned you before, accepting the senior culture decree to walk in lockstep with those who accept it puts you in a mental and emotional straightjacket. The older you get and the more immersed you are in the senior culture, the tighter the straps on the straightjacket become. They squeeze the youth-oriented attitudes and behaviors out of you. It's easy to slide into this culturally imposed straightjacket because you're conditioned to think, "All the other women my age do it. This is the way it's supposed to be."

With each passing year, the straps on the social straightjacket tighten. As the light in your eyes dims, your face and body echo what's going on in your head. Where's that youthful energy you used to project? Why is it so difficult to turn on the sparkle in your eyes? Why do you look and feel so blah? It may be that you've gotten into something that's gaining popularity: the "age gracefully" movement.

A June 14, 2007 press release titled "Neutraceutical market ripe for baby boomer products" (see www.nutraingredients-usa.com/news/ng.asp?n=77394) revealed that boomers are moving away from pharmaceuticals and toward functional foods and supplements (that's what *neutraceutical* means). Boomers are said to want to feel younger and look good for the age they're at. That's good news. So what's the bad news? According to the release, there's a strong interest in good food and proper supplements because *boomers are said to want to age gracefully.*

If you want to be ageless, deciding to "age gracefully"
is one of the most aging things you can do to yourself.

The word *graceful* is defined as kind, benevolent, benign, charming, with poise and elegance, and so on. It's a genteel word that suggests living the good life. Nursing homes are full of genteel folks who have aged gracefully. The word *reeks* of decline. You've heard the cliché "Old age is not for sissies." It's true. You enjoy or survive old age by having a well-prepared plan and a gutsy, can-do attitude that you adopt early in life. It's the antithesis of aging gracefully.

What makes me deeply cringe, however, is that the "growing old gracefully" movement finds support from influential antiaging expert Dr. Andrew Weil. He has declared that he's growing old gracefully, and his photographs reveal that he does indeed look like he's living the good life and aging gracefully. But I ask you: at sixty-three, what does he or anyone at that age know about getting old other than what is learned from books or other antiaging gurus who have yet to reach old age?

An interview with Dr. Weil was published in the *Los Angeles Times* on December 5, 2005. I bet you can imagine how I felt when I read the following:

Question: You urge people to accept the inevitability of aging. Does that mean we can't do much about it?

Weil: We can't do anything about the aging process. We cannot turn back the clock. We cannot grow younger, despite what a lot of people tell us. I think we can do a lot about remaining healthy as we get older.

Fire shot out my eyes! Dr. Weil is *completely wrong* about not being able to do anything about the aging process! Of course we can't turn back the clock, and we can't grow younger chronologically. But if preparation begins early enough in life, you can definitely manage or control the aging process, depending on how much effort you apply. Witness those of advanced years who still work, exercise, and enjoy vigorous, good health. Those people are not flukes or freaks of nature. What they enjoy is the result of hard work and determination.

By the time you're forty, you should have made the decision *not* to age traditionally. Your vision for aging should be one of strength, personal power, and independence, not wishy-washy, graceful aging.

If you adopt the desire and intent to age gracefully, I guarantee that you'll also adopt a spirit of resignation: "That's the way life is, so I'll go with the flow." An attitude of resignation and the intent to age gracefully go hand-in-hand. Both lead to uncontrolled decline.

What makes me really angry, both as an advocate for ageless aging and a pharmacist, is what Dr. Weil had to say about antiaging treatments:

Question: Has antiaging medicine (with its experimental treatments such as hormones, cellular injections, and caloric restriction to delay the aging process) produced some valuable discoveries?

Weil: No, I don't think so. [Antiaging advocates] dispense some good information about preventive health and about proper nutrition. But I think, in general, the products and services that they recommend are at best worthless and a waste of money and at worst potentially dangerous. Moreover, I think the existence of antiaging medicine is a vast distraction from what should be the important goal, which is learning how to age gracefully, how to live long and well, and how not to get sick.

His position ignores the groundbreaking work of scientist Aubrey de Grey, who maintains that we can live to at least 125 in good health by taking better care of ourselves early on, which includes eating a supernutritious but low-calorie diet. There is no question that we eat too much worthless junk, too often. As a result, we don't live as long as we could in good health because we're constantly assaulting our body with excesses that diminish its ability to handle the constant stress on vital organs.

As for hormone replacement, many midlife women need some help to achieve hormone balance. However, not all hormone replacement therapies are equal. If Dr. Weil is condemning natural bioidentical hormone therapy, he is wrong. If he's condemning synthetic hormone therapy, he is right. The chemical configuration of synthetic hormones has been altered, not so that they work better for you but so that the drug can be patented and be profitable. For example, for many years, women suffering with menopause-related problems such as hot flashes and night sweats were given a drug called Premarin that was made from the urine of pregnant mares. Women are not horses. Why should they be given synthetic, unnatural equine hormones when a natural bioidentical alternative is available? It's all about the money, ladies.

The federal government, probably with prodding by drug companies that profit from the production of synthetic hormones, is doing its best to outlaw what are known as "compounded" prescriptions of bioidentical hormone preparations. As this is written, the FDA is attempting to ban estriol, the weakest and least harmful of all estrogens in the female body. For the record, women have three types of estrogen: estriol, estrone, and estradiol. Estriol is often prescribed by antiaging physicians for vaginal dryness. Specialized pharmacies called "compounding" pharmacies prepare the doctor's order, which is personalized for the specific hormone needs of the patient. Because estriol is not patentable, drug companies make a patentable form of estradiol that doctors can prescribe. However, the weaker and safer estriol is just as effective as the stronger estradiol.

The FDA says that estriol is not an "approved drug"—even though it's natural to the female body. Why equine "conjugated estrogens" in the patented drug Premarin are "safer" than natural estrogens, I don't understand. Or maybe I do understand. If it's naturally occurring, it can't be patented. So I'll say it again: it's all about the money.

Most midlife women whose hormones have been adjusted with natural bioidentical hormone therapy will tell you how much better they feel. To suggest that natural hormone replacement is "a waste of money" and "potentially dangerous" is ludicrous. The therapy is not dangerous when prescribed by a qualified medical doctor, and it is most definitely not "fringe" medicine. The number of competent, respected physicians who prescribe natural hormone replacement therapy for their patients is testimony to the effectiveness and safety of this approach to wellness. (Books by physicians who prescribe natural hormone replacement abound in bookstores. One of my favorites is *The Miracle of Bio-Identical Hormones* by Dr. Michael E. Platt.)

To my way of thinking, Dr. Weil's goal of aging gracefully and encouraging others to follow his lead is not helpful. I wish him well and hope that he stays healthy and lives long enough to know what old age is really all about.

However, for you, know that this kind of thinking is becoming more and more pervasive. You need to maintain the necessary awareness that will help you avoid buying into the "age gracefully" movement.

As part of your awareness of all those things that can lure you down the path to the Senior Culture Club, know that more and more "experts" are going to be spouting off the same kind of nonsense spoken by Dr. Weil. Their voices are seductive, but hold your course, ladies.

Dare to be Fabulous

It's Okay to Be a Trophy

I've told you several times that appearance does not make a woman a Little Old Lady. But the reality is that every woman wants to look as good as she can for as long as she can.

I told you in the introduction that your wrinkles and gray hair do not make you a Little Old Lady. They should be the least of your worries because they are so easily fixable. But now I'm going to tackle the issue of cosmetic surgery head-on, not because it's something that is so easily done but because of our perceptions about it.

Cosmetic surgery is one of the most common and widely used antiaging tools available. However, many women would never consider going under the knife to look and feel younger. That's a perfectly valid decision; any kind of invasive surgery is not without risk. But I believe that many women don't consider cosmetic surgery because there is a stigma against it, even though it's becoming more common, especially among younger, working women. We still like to think that only self-centered movie stars and rich old ladies get face-lifts, right? Wrong.

Consider this: if you're fifty and look like sixty and feel like forty, you may be motivated to fix the outside to match how you feel inside. When you feel years younger than your actual age, it can be terribly depressing to look in the mirror each day and see an old stranger staring back at you. Seeing that image every day makes damaging self-talk run wild. "Gosh, I look so old" morphs into "I'm *really* getting old." You may want to do something in your business or personal life that requires or suggests a youthful appearance— something that's traditionally not done at your age—and the image in the mirror confirms your doubts. "Look at me; I'm too old to do that." If your appearance bothers you to that extent, it's understandable that you would want to explore your options.

If you're in an active career, an improved you will help you feel more confident. It will open up more opportunities for advancement, assuming knowledge of your age doesn't get in the way. In social situations, you'll feel (and probably will be) more accepted. If your husband or significant other tries to discourage you by saying, "I love you just the way you are," I promise that he will appreciate you even more when you look better (unless he has a control or insecurity issue).

Almost every guy would like to have a trophy wife or girlfriend to show off. When he knows he has one, his attitude and behavior can improve significantly. A relationship that's good before cosmetic surgery can become great after it. Without a doubt it's superficial, but that's the way the world turns. Remember, men are visual creatures and they like their women to look good no matter what their age.

That said, you shouldn't be a trophy for someone else. Don't get your face fixed or your teeth done for him. Sure, he gets some of the fringe benefits, but it's better to go this route when you do it to please *you*. That's what I did.

Do you remember how Cher's teeth looked when she started performing with Sonny? I'm probably the only person on earth who had the same nasty-looking teeth. But both she and I got our teeth fixed. She was young, but I was sixty-nine when I had braces put on my teeth. It became one of the best decisions I've ever made, and it didn't matter how old I was.

Now, something interesting happened about a year ago. I don't know what Cher's teeth look like today, but I'm having a problem with mine. My two front teeth began shifting inward to their original positions. My dentist recommended an orthodontist, which made me think, "Am I crazy? Why am I bothering with this?" Then I reminded myself that I continually lecture about not allowing age awareness to influence decisions you make about how you live your life. So I gave myself a mental smack on the head and made an appointment with the orthodontist. And by the way, the Invisalign process—what my orthodontist recommended for me—is painless and produces amazing results. Very briefly, the orthodontist makes a mold of your mouth and then creates a series of lightweight, painless forms called appliances. Depending on how much adjustment needs to be done, you wear each appliance for about a month or until the desired result is reached.

Six years ago I decided to have my face "fixed." I had a face-lift and my ears pinned back. To this day I am happy I did it. When I look in the mirror, the person looking back at me reflects the person I am on the inside—the "real" me. Before the procedure, my husband assured me that he loved me just the way I was and said I looked fabulous. (Love is blind.) Before I had braces, he insisted that he never noticed my crooked teeth. But he loves my new smile. He now says that when he looks at me, it makes him feel younger, and that makes us both feel good. As one old geezer passed us on the street, he whispered to my husband, "It must be nice to have a young wife." Yes, it's shallow, it's nauseating, but that's the way it is!

If you decide to undergo a cosmetic procedure, use caution. Thoroughly check the credentials and reputation of any cosmetic surgeon before you sign on. And please don't expect perfection. Cosmetic surgery is an art, not a science. Be sure to examine the surgeon's portfolio of before-and-after pictures; they tell a lot about a surgeon's skill if you look carefully enough. For example, how well the surgeon performs on eyes will show up consistently. I recall one cosmetic surgeon I interviewed who talked a great game, but his portfolio told a slightly different story. Also understand that only the best before-and-after photos make it into the album. Moreover, some unscrupulous surgeons may put photos of other surgeons' work in their own portfolios and pass it off as their own. Finally, and very importantly, check the doctor's status with your state medical board (go to www.ama-assn.org/ama/pub/category/2645.html for links to state medical boards). Also check your local court records to see whether the doctor has been sued. One place to begin your search is at http://searchenginez.com/courtrecords_usa.html. Be as informed as you can possibly be. For more insight, please read Susan Gail's book, *Cosmetic Surgery: Before, Between and After.*

Conscientious surgeons will be happy to thoroughly discuss possible risks with you. They want to make sure you understand what you're getting into, so pay attention so you can make an educated decision. By the way, I don't recommend choosing an inexpensive surgeon in Mexico or any place outside the United States. What recourse would you have if the surgery turned out badly? Would you be able to go back for fixes—assuming fixes would be possible? This is one time you don't shop around for the best price; you want competence. A bad outcome can be as life changing as a good outcome, so weigh your decision carefully.

If you decide you want to fix your face but are discouraged by the expense, look at it two ways:

- Recall how much money you've wasted on cosmetic products over the years (and continue to waste) that haven't produced the results they promise in advertising.

- You can pay for cosmetic procedures the same as you do a car—that is, over time. Both will depreciate over time, but your face will look better longer than any car.

This discussion is not to encourage you to have cosmetic surgery. No one should tell you what you should or should not do. Elective surgery is a very personal decision, with risks as well as rewards. If you have the slightest doubt and aren't convinced it's the right thing to do, then don't do it!

If you remain skeptical about cosmetic surgery, that's okay. Some women like their wrinkles, and I've always maintained that wrinkles don't make you old or less attractive—or a Little Old Lady; your mind-set and lifestyle do that. I've met many beautiful older women with less-than-flawless skin who will never, ever become Little Old Ladies. How do I know this? Because they have unleashed the pit bull within them, and that will keep them youthful forever.

If you do decide to upgrade your appearance by whatever means and to whatever extent, before you do anything else, improve your smile. I've already touched on the importance of a nice smile, but I need to elaborate on it. On an older face, little gives the appearance of advanced age more than yellow teeth. Or worse, brown teeth. Get your teeth whitened if you can. There are new techniques being developed all the time to whiten teeth, and the process is well worth investigating. If your teeth need straightening or replacing, go for it. As I've already mentioned, the Invisalign procedure to straighten teeth is painless and produces amazing results.

Picture this: a face that has been lifted or had its wrinkles lasered away, but with a smile that reveals brown or yellow teeth. A face that looks thirty-something will look bizarre with a smile that reveals old-looking teeth.

Another important reason to fix your teeth first is that more than 75 percent of all older people have infected gums to some extent, according to the University of Maryland Medical Center website (see http://searchenginez.com/courtrecords_usa.html). This is a serious health issue. Bacteria from a low-grade infection in the gums circulate continuously throughout the body, from the top of your head to your feet. The result can be headaches, achy joints, a lack of energy, and a host of other health problems that seem to have no cause. *First things first when it comes to improving your appearance!*

My Skin Story

There is another important thing I haven't touched on: controlling the effect of the aging process on your skin. The cosmetics market is flooded with every conceivable type of antiaging product. Many of them are good, and every woman has her favorite. It's interesting that what works for one woman often does not work for another. What follows is my story.

I have been blessed with great skin. It's smooth and unwrinkled. I have some lines across my forehead and between my eyes, and that's about it. I should be at least somewhat wrinkled, and my skin should have that dried, cross-hatched appearance that is typical of older skin. Clearly I'm an older woman, but my skin says I'm a lot younger than my chronological age. People on the street stop and ask me what I use. I remember going into a McDonald's once and a woman immediately stopped me and asked what I used on my face.

So what's the deal?

I assume that heredity has something to do with it, but remember, many gerontologists are in agreement: how well you age is 70 percent the result of lifestyle choices that you make early on in your life and only 30 percent the result of heredity.

I believe this is why my skin looks as good as it does. For years I've taken megadoses of Vitamin C in the form of calcium ascorbate. (I talk more about this in Strategy No. 13.) Vitamin C supports formation of collagen, which keeps the skin young and firm. In addition, I use prescription Retin-A. (More about Retin A in Strategy No. 13.) Retin-A is not for everyone, and it must be used carefully, but it works for me. Finally, I drink a lot of water. If you don't stay hydrated, your skin will reflect the lack of internal moisture. Please don't make the mistake of thinking that everything liquid is hydrating—it's not. Coffee and alcohol are dehydrating. Colas and soft drinks in general are poison for your skin. Just as a recap, this is why you need eight to ten eight-ounce glasses of pure, unfluoridated water every day:

It is essential for digestion and nutrient absorption and elimination.

- It aids your circulation.
- It helps control your body's temperature.
- It lubricates and cushions your joints.
- It keeps your skin healthy.
- It helps remove toxins from your body.

Whatever you decide to do to improve your appearance, know that the results can add happy years to how you feel. You're not vain to do it, either. You want to look good no matter how old you are. If you're doing the work to keep your body and your mind in shape, then it stands to reason that you do the things that can help improve your facial appearance as well.

Lastly, it's a fact of life that the first thing people see is your face. In the first three seconds of meeting you, they make a decision about your age, competence, health, and mental status. If making the right impression is important to you, if it will make you feel better to have the face you had ten or more years ago, it's your right. After carefully considering all the factors involved, feel free to have a face that reflects how you feel and function, regardless of the number of years you've lived.

Unleash Your Pit Bull

Challenge and Keep Your Physical Capacity

A s you age, maintaining mental and physical health, strength, and flexibility is paramount. I've talked at length about the importance of continuing to focus on your mental "future image." I've given you different strategies to help you maintain the right mental attitude about your age. Now I'm going to spend some time giving you my approach to keeping your body in as good as shape as your mind. In this strategy and the next, I'm going to talk about diet and exercise. And by the way, if your weight is an issue, there is no magic pill that will take it off—never has been, never will be, no matter what the commercials try to sell you. What will take off the weight is eating an antiaging diet and living an energetic, antiaging lifestyle that includes regular exercise.

I won't kid you—getting and staying healthy takes effort! Any worthwhile food and exercise program will tell you that while it can give you the tools you need to look and feel healthy, it all comes down to your determination. You need to decide to do it and then *do it.*

Once you make a firm decision to eat well and exercise consistently, be aware that things will happen that conspire against your progress. You will backslide, as everyone does. But with the right attitude, it doesn't matter. If life puts a roadblock in your way, it doesn't matter; you will find a way around it. If you stumble, you will pick yourself up and start over. So be prepared for difficulties. Know that they are going to be there, so be determined to forge ahead in spite of them. Anything worth having is worth working for. *The payoff comes when you are old in years but young in mind and body. The outcome is so phenomenal, it is worth whatever sweat you put into it.*

Take Stock of What You Got

Where do you begin? You start by taking an inventory of your present physical competencies. What are you able to do now that you always want to be able to do? Everyone has his or her own unique list of priorities.

For me, being able to move quickly and with assurance has always been a priority. In observing old people, walking briskly is something they often can't do. It's a sign of decline and a handicap. There are times when, whatever your age, you simply have to get out of the way and do it fast. I stay aware of what I must do to continue to move quickly and with good posture. To help me do that, my trusty treadmill is one of my best friends.

What about you? Can you still walk at a brisk pace? If that's important to you, what will you do to make certain you don't lose that ability? Are you determined enough to walk every day on a treadmill or in a safe place outside to maintain an energetic stride? Young people move confidently. It's effortless for them. They don't have to think about their agility. A young person capable of performing any youthful skill doesn't stop and think, "Unless I work at keeping this skill, I will eventually lose it." That doesn't happen because young people don't need to make conscious decisions about what or how they do something; they have the gift of youth. Unfortunately, youth has the capacity to con you into believing it will be around forever. Furthermore, it gives no warning other than overlooked visual cues that it is slipping away. Your youth doesn't care what happens to you after it leaves, either.

However, there comes a time as you age when you start to lose that effortless agility. The key is to stay in shape so that there is a smooth transition between the time when youthful agility is taken for granted and the time when youthful agility is the result of conscious effort. You want your physical ability to stay as seamless as possible. Remember, your existence manager doesn't want you to keep what you have—it wants to get you to the finish line on its schedule.

It's not the passage of time that matters but how time and effort are managed during the passage!

When was the last time you could bend and touch your toes? Can you still climb a flight of stairs without getting out of breath? Can you hold yourself upright, or are you tilting toward the floor, not because of osteoporosis but because of inattentiveness to your posture? When you shop at the market, do you lean on your basket as you push it along, not because your back hurts but because you are tired or careless? Tired and careless are not acceptable excuses. Stay aware and straighten up!

Start to work to keep your inventoried physical, youthful talents that you have today. If you can bend and touch your toes now, then keep doing it regularly. Preferably daily. If you don't do it, one day you'll try to bend over to tie your shoes and you won't be able to. Then you'll tell yourself, "I must be getting old." Suggestion: if you can bend and only get as far as your knees, enroll in a yoga or exercise class to help you stay strong and flexible and manage how your body ages.

Youth Is Slippery—Pay Attention to Its Departure Signs

Regrettably, at some point after age thirty, youth doesn't tap you on the shoulder and say, "Hey babe, I've given you thirty to forty good years. I'm tired of being abused and taken for granted. I'm leaving—you need to take over and fend for yourself. But because we've been together so long, I won't desert you all at once. I'll leave gradually to give you a chance to set up a program to help you keep what I've given you. But frankly my dear, I don't think you have the guts to do it."

Even though you haven't heard youth whisper that message into your ear, if you are over thirty, assume that youth has delivered that message. How do you react? Your response to the inaudible but clear challenge should be "Okay, I hear you. Thank you for the warning. But no guts? Just watch me!"

Without your being aware, youth slowly hands over its control to your existence manager, whose job is to lead you to your final destination. If you understand that this is the path of the aging process, you are in a position of power. You can do what conventional wisdom says can't be done!

When you slack off on staying fit and eating properly, when you neglect controllable aspects of aging, you don't see immediate results. Nothing seems to have changed. (Again, that's how youth cons you into inactivity.) You see little or nothing to remind you that unless you make a conscious effort to maintain the youthful characteristics, attributes, and skills that you take for granted, *you will lose them.*

You can't hire someone to get inside your head and tell you what to do every day. You are the boss of what's in your head, so act like you're the boss and take control!

We aren't designed to live forever, but if you attempt to take control of your mind and body, then you can live more fully for as long as you live; you won't just exist. You can maintain a strong, healthy, supple body and a sharp, flexible mind far longer than traditionally considered the norm—regardless of how much your existence manager tries to drag you in the opposite direction.

Right now, if you haven't done so already, inventory your youthful skills and attributes. Pinpoint physical competencies that you want to keep or improve as you age, and devise a plan to make it happen. You can't stop all change, but you can moderate much of it. Effort pays off.

Always push yourself. If you think you have pushed yourself as hard as you can, then push some more if you can do so without injuring yourself. Be a pit bull with yourself. If you don't make yourself do what you should do, who will do it for you?

How do you win the power struggle with your existence manager? The answer is to take control of your being by declaring, "I will do whatever it takes to keep what I have right now." Then you just do it, even if life tosses you a curve ball now and then. No excuses.

Trying to control your existence manager doesn't mean that you'll keep the same outward facial or physical appearance for the next twenty-five years, but that really doesn't matter. You know that cosmetic procedures can now make you look any way you choose. What cosmetic surgery can do for your face, you can do for your body with regular exercise. However, no cosmetic procedure or product on the market will maintain your inner body in a perpetually healthy, youthful condition. That's up to you to accomplish with the diet and lifestyle choices you make—starting now.

Perpetual Awareness Is Key

Caution: don't decide to be ageless only on your birthday or when the thought pops into your head. Don't do it only when you look in the mirror and suddenly notice serious signs of decline. That's as good as doing nothing.

I've said it before, and it's important enough to say again: put perpetual awareness in the forefront of your consciousness, and make it a driving force in your life. You can't change or manage what you're not aware of. Be assured that to do so is neither a burden nor an obsession. It becomes an instinctive part of your daily life, part of who you are and how you live. Once you internalize the question "What can I control about my aging process and how can I do it," then antiaging thinking and behaviors go on automatic pilot. Knowing what you want for yourself tomorrow becomes infused in how you live today. It eventually pays off in ways you cannot imagine now.

Bad things do happen to good people who do all the right things. How do you control that reality? You can't, but you can come to terms with it and do the best you can. That's the way life is. But if you make an attempt to control your aging process while you're in good health, you *will* deal with fewer negative things that are traditionally and *mistakenly* believed to be the result of old age.

This Is What Matters Most

A Healthy Mind and *Body*

In order for you to keep that tight leash on your existence manager, you must stay as healthy as you possibly can. I have yet to see a Little Old Lady whose health is in tiptop condition. Your health depends on your mind-set, lifestyle, what you put into your mouth in terms of food and supplements, and how willing you are to exercise. You can do it. And it's easier than you've been led to believe.

To what degree do you make your health a priority? For example, do you take at least a multiple vitamin on a daily basis, without fail? If you're like a lot of people, even though you know you should take better care of yourself, your existence manager is not rooting for your healthy longevity. It constantly tries to sabotage your best efforts. When you want to make your health a primary concern, it whispers, "It's okay, sweetie. You don't have to take your vitamins today." So you don't take your vitamins today, and you probably forget about taking them the next day, the next week, and the next month. Your existence manager also does a great job of helping you brush off guilt. For example, when you are about to order a double cheeseburger at the fast-food restaurant, it whispers, "Forget about the fat and the calories. One more burger isn't going to kill you. Life is short. Enjoy it." *Stay in charge of your existence manager!* If you don't take care of yourself, who will? (I know I keep harping on this, but it's important!)

Consider the following sobering information: In 2003, a study funded by Wyeth Consumer Healthcare showed that daily use of a multivitamin by older adults could lead to more than $1.6 billion in Medicare savings over the next five years. The study, the first of its kind, included a systematic literature review of the most rigorous research available and examined the health effects of multivitamin use among adults over sixty-five years of age. Over the five-year period from 2004–2008, the study results showed potential savings from a reduction in hospitalizations for heart attacks, as well as Medicare nursing home stays and home healthcare-associated infection. Researchers also reviewed literature that examined the preventive benefits of multivitamin supplementation as it relates to colorectal cancer, prostate cancer, diabetes, and osteoporosis. (See resources for the Wyeth Report link.)

If we can't even take a multivitamin every day, clearly we are not getting the motivation we need to stay healthy. The Wyeth report is compelling evidence that something in our society doesn't work in the best interests of our aging population. Since this report was issued in 2003, has the government, the drug companies, or any influential entity consistently urged older people to take at least one daily supplement? Has your physician urged you to take a daily supplement? Has there been a mass movement to implement the low-cost, money-saving findings of this study? Sure, vitamins are shown on TV, but that's just advertising. Where are the authoritative voices to validate the need for at least a daily supplement? Many people won't take a supplement without first asking their doctor, whose knowledge of nutrition may be lacking.

If you haven't done so already, find a qualified, traditionally trained physician with expertise in antiaging medicine and nutrition. He or she will help you rethink your relationship with food and medicine. This is a priority!

You can reach your health goals without the help of an antiaging physician, but you may find it difficult on your own. An antiaging physician who understands natural hormone replacement therapy, natural insulin management, and dietary supplements can get your body in balance so that you burst with energy and enjoy being disease-free, in good spirits, and in control of your weight. (To find an antiaging physician in your area, visit the American College for Advancement of Medicine website at www.ACAM.org.)

Educate Yourself about Antiaging Nutrition

An antiaging physician (also known as an alternative or integrative physician) will give you plenty of guidance, but you are responsible for informing yourself. *Your doctor can't and shouldn't do everything for you.*

Bookstore shelves are loaded with titles that offer great nutrition and antiaging lifestyle information. With a bit of investigation, you'll discover that the Internet is awash with websites that can teach you everything you need to know about diet and nutrition. However, if you're a total newbie to nutrition and supplementation, use caution when starting your research on the Internet. It's often difficult to recognize which sites are trustworthy. I recommend beginning with Dr. Joseph Mercola's site (www.mercola.com), which is known for its reliable and comprehensive information. Dr. Mercola is an osteopathic physician who operates the Optimal Wellness Center in Hoffman Estates, Illinois. Be aware that his site is also loaded with advertisements, but the health information is top notch.

Also trustworthy is the Life Extension Foundation site (www.lef.org), which also publishes *Life Extension* magazine. I like the magazine because the well-documented articles are written by knowledgeable, health-oriented writers, researchers, and physicians. The foundation also sells supplements and other health-related items to support longevity research. See the resources section at the end of this book for suggestions on print newsletters written by alternative physicians as well as a list of books to read. Check with nutrition-orientated friends who are doing well. What are they reading?

This Is What Works for Me

My own antiaging program is basic and uncomplicated. I eat simply, meaning chicken, eggs, vegetables, nuts, whole-grain bread and cereals, and some fruit. I mix butter with olive oil to make a soft spread. I use bran and psyllium to hopefully stave off colon cancer. I consume a lot of fluoride-free water. I eat very little fish because so much of it is farmed and contaminated with mercury. (I use certified, pure salmon oil.) When you look at farmed salmon in the supermarket seafood case, you will probably be impressed by the bright pink color. Fish farmers use a chemical in the unnatural feed the fish are fed to produce the appealing pink color (see "Issues of Purity and Pollution Leave Farmed Salmon Looking Less Rosy," *The New York Times*, June 2008).

No fancy cooking for me, either. I like to say that I gave up my love affair with food a long time ago, but the truth is I never had an affair with food. I eat to live, not the other way around, and what a blessing it is that I'm able to do that. Cravings and a ravenous appetite do not torture me. I am liberated to eat what I know is good for me, although I must admit that I love McDonald's. A word in defense of fast food: I believe it's not all as terribly bad as we are led to believe. Yes, it's overloaded with grease, calories, and trans fats, but the menus are much more diverse than they used to be. You have choices!

It's up to you to use common sense when you order fast food. For example, I would never order fries, a Big Mac, or Chicken McNuggets. But McDonald's and its rivals now offer a variety of salads. By choosing a low-calorie dressing, you can have a decent meal. Or you can order a fish sandwich and scrape off the excess mayonnaise. Of course you shouldn't order soda, diet or otherwise, to wash down your meal—it's all loaded with chemicals that aren't good for you, and it has an unbelievable amount of sodium. In the end, it's a matter of exercising good judgment. The less often you frequent a fast food place, the better off you are. The more fresh fruits and veggies, whole grains, and lean meats you eat, the better. But then, you probably already know that!

Free Radicals and the Aging Process

Many theories abound about what causes aging, but the one that appeals to me most is the free radical theory. Basically, this theory says that aging is caused by activity of "free radicals." Free radicals result from the breakdown of food and drink, environmental pollutants such as cigarettes and pesticides, and also from just living and breathing. Free radicals are unavoidable. Chemically they are molecules that are very unstable because they do not have an even number of electrons. They want to be stable, so they always look for an extra electron they can steal from a healthy molecule to become stable. In the scavenging process to gain stability, the electrons they steal turn healthy cells, each with a missing electron, into free radicals. This snowball effect causes damage to healthy tissue in the form of aging or the start of a disease process.

The good news is that substances called antioxidants can help control free radicals. Antioxidants are found in fruits and vegetables, and the body can also make some of them. Antioxidants keep free radicals in your body from making your cells old. The problem is that most people don't eat enough antioxidant-rich food, and they don't take antioxidant supplements to make up for the deficiency. Most antiaging experts—including scientist Dr. Aubrey de Grey, chairman and chief science officer of the Methuselah Foundation (www.mfoundation.org/index. php?pagename=mf_who)—agree that protecting the cells in your body from free radical damage is key to controlling the aging process.

My thinking is that even if you adhere to a strict antiaging diet, you can't get enough antioxidants from food alone. If in addition to a nutritious diet, you also take medications, beware; many medications are notorious for depleting nutrients. For example, statins, which many people take to lower cholesterol, deplete CoQ10, an antioxidant that is vital for a healthy heart. (See "Coenzyme Q10, Lipid-Lowering Drugs [Statins] and Cholesterol: A Present Day Pandora's Box" by Dr. Emile G. Bliznakov at www.ana-jana.org/reprints/CoQ10Reprint.pdf.)

When you consider that our food supply comes from all over the world, you have to wonder about the quality of the soil in which food is grown; what kind of fertilizers, pesticides, and other chemicals are used; and the length of shipping time, as well as storage conditions along the way. When you can keep a bunch of asparagus from Chile in your refrigerator for two weeks (as I've done, having forgotten about it) and the stalks remain as fresh looking as the day they were harvested, you have to assume that something is wrong. It's not natural for fresh food to stay fresh so long. What chemicals have been used to extend their shelf life?

When tomatoes in the supermarket are all uniformly red, that's not natural. At what stage of ripening were they gassed to produce such uniform color? Does it ever bother you that the produce departments of most supermarkets are so picture-perfect? Whatever do they do to fruit and vegetables to keep them in such pristine condition? You get what I'm saying, right? Unless your fruits and veggies are free of pesticides and other harmful chemicals you run the risk of putting as many or more bad things into your body than good things. And even organic fruits and veggies run the risk of being nutrient deficient because the soil used to grow them may be depleted.

This Is My Routine

Because I don't rely on food alone, I spend a lot of money on supplements. Basically, my list is heavy with antioxidants. Here it is, although it's not complete and is subject to change:

- Alpha lipoic acid
- Alpha lipoic acid Acetyl-L-carnitine
- Alpha lipoic acid N-acetyl cysteine
- Alpha lipoic acid Vitamin C in various forms, but primarily calcium ascorbate, which I rely on for calcium

- Alpha lipoic acid Vitamin E (mixed tocopherols and tocotrienols)
- Alpha lipoic acid Coenzyme Q10
- Alpha lipoic acid Fish oil capsules and salmon oil
- Alpha lipoic acid High-potency B complex
- Alpha lipoic acid Hyaluronic acid capsules
- Alpha lipoic acid Vitamin D3
- Alpha lipoic acid Assortment of other antioxidants, including curcumin, ginkgo biloba, astaxanthin, grapeseed, resveratrol, and SAM-e

As the TV commercial says, "But wait, there's more!"

Yes, there is a lot more. To elaborate, first thing in the morning before breakfast I take my "wakeup potion" that consists of calcium ascorbate crystals, collagen powder, a potent greens powder, flaxseed meal, fruit, water, and orange juice. I use this potion to wash down my major supplements.

Why this mixture? I take calcium ascorbate crystals, a nonacidic form of vitamin C, because it's easy on the stomach, tasteless, and soluble in water. I take about ten grams (10,000 milligrams) at a time. The government has established that the minimum daily requirement for vitamin C is around fifty milligrams. That's about all you would get in a glass of orange juice. That amount, although better than nothing, doesn't help control the ravages of aging.

I use collagen powder to help support bones and joints and, above all, to keep my skin smooth. Collagen also keeps my fingernails hard. Cosmetic creams that are supposed to promote collagen production are rather useless in my opinion. Smear as much stuff on your face as you like, but good skin comes from the inside out. I also take hyaluronic acid capsules for my skin. The one exception to my inside-out rule is prescription Retin-A cream, which I've already mentioned. It really works to smooth the surface of the skin.

I believe using a potent greens powder is essential to keep your body in an alkaline state. It would be better to juice my own fresh greens, but I don't have time. The other reason I use a greens powder is that it's almost impossible to eat enough nutritious green vegetables. Eating a serving of broccoli or spinach grown in deficient soil treated with chemicals to extend shelf life and sprayed with pesticides does little to enhance health. As I've said, I can't count on daily intake of vegetables or fruit to provide enough nutrients to maintain and protect health. I simply can't eat that much. I don't think anyone can.

On Being Alkaline

Why is it important for your body to be on the alkaline side rather than the acidic? I believe that cancer can't survive in an alkaline environment. If you wonder how acidic or alkaline your body is, go to the health food store or a pharmacy and purchase test strips to determine the balance. Put a strip on your tongue. If you are in an alkaline state, the paper turns green. That's an ideal state for your body to be in. If it turns yellow, you are in an acidic state. A yellowish-greenish color, somewhere in the middle, is okay but not ideal. The greener the color, the more alkaline your body is, and that's what you want to shoot for. Keeping the body alkaline is not complicated.

The chart that follows shows which foods are acid, alkaline, and in-between. I believe it is generally agreed that your diet should be 75 percent alkaline and 25 percent acid (see www.alive.com/4387a12a2.php?subject_bread_cramb=188). Foods from the alkaline columns are generally higher in antiaging antioxidants. Which foods from which column do you consume most often? Now is the time to rethink and retool your diet!

	Most Alkaline	Medium Alkaline	Low Alkaline	Food Categories	Low Acid	Medium Acid	Most Acid
1							
2	baking soda	spices/ cinnamon	most herbs	Seasonings	curry	vanilla / nutmeg	jam / jelly
3							
4	cantaloupe	apple	orange		dried fruit	plum	cranberry
5	honeydew	avocado	apricot		fig	prune	pomegranate
6	lime	cherry	banana	Fruits	raisin	tomato	
7	nectarine	grapefruit	blueberry		date		
8	raspberry	lemon	papaya				
9	water-melon	mango	pineapple				
10	tangerine	pear	grape				
11		peach	strawberry				
12							
13	broccoli	bell pepper	Brussels sprouts		carrots	chard	carob
14	collard greens	cauli-flower	beet	Vegetables	corn on cob	chickpeas	peanut butter
15	daikon radish	eggplant	cabbage		rhubarb	green peas	processed soy beans

16	garlic	kohlrabi	chive	**Beans**	kidney beans	lima beans	
17	kale	parsnip	dark lettuce		spinach	navy beans	
18	lentils	endive	mushroom	**Legumes**	string beans	peanuts	
19	onion	mustard greens	potato			pinto beans	
20	parsley	ginger root	pumpkin			white beans	
21	sea vegetables	sweet potato	squash			tofu	
22							
23		almonds	avocado oil	**Nuts / Seeds**	almond oil	cashews	brazil nuts
24		cod liver oil	coconut oil		canola oil	pecans	hazelnuts
25		poppy seeds	flax oil	**Sprouts**	grape-seed oil	pistachios	walnuts
26		primrose oil	olive oil		green soybeans	sesame	
27			sesame seeds	**Oils**	pine nuts	sunflower oil	
28			sprouts		pumpkin seed oil		
29							
30			oats	**Grains**	brown rice	corn	barley
31			quinoa		buckwheat	rye	
32			wild rice	**Cereals**	kasha	oat bran	
33					millet	wheat	
34							
35				**Fish**	fish	chicken	beef
36					turkey	lamb	lobster
37				**Fowl**	venison	pork	
38					wild duck	shellfish	
39						veal	
40							
41				**Dairy / Eggs**	chicken eggs	cows' milk	processed cheese
42			quail eggs		cream	soy cheese	ice cream
43					yogurt	fresh cheese	
44							
45		green tea	ginger tea	**Beverages**	Kona coffee	black tea	coffee
46							beer

47							
48		molasses	rice syrup	Sweeteners	honey	saccharin	sugar
49					maple syrup		cocoa
50		apple cider vinegar			rice vinegar	balsamic vinegar	white vinegar

If you want to know all the supplements I take (the list is subject to change), they're in Art Linkletter's and Mark Victor Hansen's book *How to Make the Rest of Your Life the Best of Your Life.*

If you aren't taking supplements, you don't have to start with what's on my list. In fact, I don't recommend that you do. Start with a good, daily multivitamin such as Centrum or other brand of your choice. Take as recommended on the container label. As you become more informed, you'll want to add other supplements to your daily regimen and adjust dosages. I encourage you to consider the excellent books and newsletters in the resources section. It's not enough to know what anyone else takes. It's important to educate yourself and find out what makes sense for you.

Strategy No. 14:

You Must Have a Regimen!

The Fast-Food System to
Control Your Aging Process

In order to take your vitamins and other necessary antiaging supplements, in order to maintain your health and be in charge of your aging process, you must have a plan that includes a daily "do or die" regimen. It is absolutely vital. To stay truly ageless you must have the right mindset, get the right nutrition, exercise, and sleep—preferably without the aid of any drug. All of this must be so automatic that discussions with yourself about "should I or shouldn't I do it today" or "do I have time today" just don't happen. You have the attitude to "just do it." That's one of my major rules for successfully managing the aging process. *Just do what you know you have to do.* And to do that you need to establish a regimen.

What is a regimen? It's any system you devise that helps you maintain and improve your health on a daily basis. It should also be simple enough that you can stick with it, so that you can be where you want your health and life to be in twenty-five years.

How do you develop such a system? As I suggested at the beginning of this book, think McDonald's. If you eat fast food even occasionally, you have to admire how quickly the workers crank out the products. A proven, time-tested system makes this speed possible. Every day they prepare and serve every burger and every batch of fries exactly the same way; no deviation from is the system allowed. It works perfectly except when humans goof up and don't follow the system.

- The fast-food system teaches a lot about mastering the aging process if you apply it to your own life. The system goes like this:

- Start with a product (you).

- Develop a lifestyle system or regimen (exercise, diet, and proper mind-set) to maintain and improve the product (you).

- Apply your lifestyle system to the product (you).

- Do it the same way every day.

Simple, isn't it?

Let's assume you decide that your system includes seven basic actions you'll take each and every day to help you stay ageless. For example:

1. You eat breakfast with enough protein to keep your appetite in check until the next meal. No sugary, fake cereals or excess empty carbs to upset your blood sugars that in turn make you feel shaky and have cravings.

2. You take vitamin supplements, even if you feel great and think you don't need them. (If you believe you

don't need supplements, your existence manager is in charge—not you! Remember, its job is to hasten your arrival at your final destination on its timeline, not yours.)

3. You make time to exercise, even if you think you don't have time. No need for trips to a fitness center; instead, invest in a treadmill or stationary bike and put it in front of the TV. Walk or pedal away while you watch your favorite programs instead of sitting on the sofa drinking fattening (yes, fattening) diet soda and wolfing down bags of greasy chips. (See "Study: Artificial Sweeteners Increase Weight Gain Odds," *ABC News*, February 11, 2008.)

This is important: It doesn't matter if you don't like to exercise—develop a routine and stick with it. (Check with your physician before starting an exercise program.) I don't like to exercise. There are times—lots of times—when I would prefer to sit and vegetate. But this is where my fierce inner pit bull, Rocky, springs into action. (I introduced you to him in Strategy No. 2.) I have trained him so that when I think I'd rather sit he snarls, "Barbara, get off your butt, and get on the treadmill." I listen to Rocky because I know the price I will pay if I don't exercise. I have that clear vision in my mind of what I want to look and feel like "forever," and it's more powerful than the lure of a cushy chair and my existence manager trying to drag me to the finish line sooner than I care to reach it.

Please understand that I'm not advocating that you exercise and diet to the point that you're model thin. If you're that way naturally, that's fine. However, to make yourself that thin is actually not healthy. What we're aiming for here is a healthy weight, muscle strength, and a toned body. That's the condition I'm in. I'm size 8-10, and as along as I can fit into clothes that size, I don't worry about my weight.

4.   You spend at least fifteen minutes reading books or newsletters that teach you about antiaging nutrition and healthy living. (See the resources section for suggestions.)

5.   You drink eight eight-ounce glasses of water during the day. If there is fluoride in your water, invest in a filter to remove it. A quick check on the Internet will provide a massive amount of credible information that explains why mass medication with fluoride is dangerous. In chemistry class in pharmacy school, I can still see the professor explaining why fluoride is so toxic. One compelling argument against water fluoridation comes from dentist David C. Kennedy in a letter to the Santa Cruz, California Board of Supervisors (see www.nofish.org/new_page_17. htm). The most effective way to remove fluoride is by reverse osmosis. You can install a system under your kitchen sink that will do the job. The water will taste flat, but adding some calcium ascorbate crystals will improve the taste.

6.   You get seven to eight hours of sleep every night.

7.   Learn to manage your stress. If something irritates you today, ask yourself if what you are stressing out about will even be a memory next week. If stress is a relentless ogre in your life, please read *Bless Your Stress* by C. Leslie Charles and Mimi Donaldson. Despite the serious nature of this topic, I promise that *Bless Your Stress* will make you nod in agreement, smile in amusement, and maybe even laugh out loud. This book will help you discover how you unknowingly create and maybe even perpetuate your stress. If anything can help break the stress cycle, this book is it.

Just Do It!

It's a no-brainer: you consistently do the seven actions of your choice each day. If you already have incorporated these steps into a daily regime, well done! You are well on your way to living an ageless life, with all of its joys and benefits. I bet that many of you are doing at least some of the above steps already—and I congratulate you, too. Just make sure to incorporate the others into your daily regimen. If you don't do all of the steps at once, don't despair and please don't feel overwhelmed.

In Ben Franklin's autobiography, he listed twelve attributes that he wanted to emulate—but he also knew himself. He knew that trying to do all twelve would have stopped him from doing even one. So, he wrote that he would work on one attribute a week, starting with the first one, and adding one each week until he had them all down pat.

You can be like Ben. You don't need to start all seven steps at once. Start with just one—the easiest one for you to do. Do it until it becomes a habit, until it doesn't matter if the sky falls—*you do it anyway*. Then, after the first action becomes a habit, add another. If you are thirty, forty, or fifty and begin to invest in yourself with a dedicated system that makes sense, I guarantee that by the time you're seventy-nine (my age), Mother Time will have no claim on your ageless life. You'll feel and function as well (or better) than you did twenty-five years earlier. You will never be a Little Old Lady.

Looking Ahead: Prepare for Life on Your Own

How to Survive When the Love of Your Life Is Gone

Well, my friends, you now know all that I know about how to avoid becoming a Little Old Lady. I work on my mind-set every day, just as I walk each night on my treadmill for thirty minutes and use my Gazelle for thirty minutes. (If you watch enough TV, you know that a Gazelle is not an animal but a type of exercise equipment.) I take my nutritional supplements every morning. I follow my regimen. In other words, I just do what I know I have to do.

However, there is one point that I must address because it has come up time and time again in my workshops and seminars and from people seeking help. It's not the most pleasant topic to think about, and many of us shy away from it because it can be so painful. Here it is: if you're married or in a committed relationship, you'd be wise to do some mental preparation for the loss of your loved one. You don't have to be old or older for it to happen; it can happen when you least expect it.

Losing your loved one, especially when it's sudden, can wreck havoc on your emotional health—and not in the way that you think. It's devastating to lose your partner, the person you have loved, cherished, fought and then made up with for however many years. It can be extremely aging mentally and physically. But, while many good books and support groups are out there to help you through the grieving process, no one likes to talk about what happens after you've said good-bye and handled the personal effects.

In a recent article for my newsletter titled "Prepare to Survive a Curve Ball," I discuss what to do when the love of your life is gone. After the article was published, I received an email from a woman I'll call Luann who had recently suffered the loss of her husband. I'm including her response here because it is so instructive:

> Barbara, I think you are right on. When I was teaching high school, I felt young and attractive. Now that I have retired and especially now that I am recently widowed, I feel old, useless, and not wanted. A widow becomes a fifth wheel: never invited into the circle of friends you had when you were a couple. When going to group dinners, singles are placed at tables off by themselves. I am now dealing with both age and being without the love of my life and escort. I go to lunch often with other widows (my age). I work in three volunteer organizations, but all involve old people. I have just finished reading the book *How to Make the Rest of Your Life the Best of Your Life*. Many suggestions

require money and a companion, neither of which I have. HELP. Any other good suggestions? Luann

In summary, this is Luann's dilemma:

- She's retired, widowed, and lonely.
- She has no plans for the future.
- She wants social interaction but not with "old" people.
- She volunteers, but it's not fulfilling.
- She could use more income.

These are all the typical problems that arise when a person loses his or her beloved life partner. What struck me first about Luann's situation was that she didn't have enough money to do the things she'd like to do. I constantly advise against healthy, financially strapped retirees spending time volunteering when they should be earning a paycheck. Luann's situation validates my position. It is unfortunate when mentally and physically able retirees struggle and do without for lack of satisfying employment that would enhance their quality of life.

Of course, I'm not opposed to volunteering. Many worthy organizations rely on volunteers to get their work done. For those who are financially secure, volunteering gets them back into the real world, helps broaden their outlook, and raises their self-esteem. But I'm clearly on the side of employment. Nothing beats getting a paycheck every week—even if you don't "need" it.

There's also a wealth of information that rests underneath Luann's actual words. She writes, "When I was teaching high school, I felt young and attractive. Now that I have retired and especially now that I am recently widowed, I feel old, useless, and not wanted." This tells me that she felt young and attractive while working because it associated her with young, attractive, mentally stimulating coworkers. Their youth and vitality helped nourish and support her perception of her own youth and vitality. This is why I keep harping on the value of associating with younger people as well as people your own age. Luann speaks about often having lunch with other same-age widows. A pleasant pastime, but ultimately, one that is aging and depressing.

Because I don't know why she retired, I can't comment on her decision. But I do know this: *Luann should have had a strategy for life after retirement, including a plan for what she could do if she was suddenly left alone.*

Clearly, Luann didn't prepare for her husband's demise. While he was alive, she did what most women do: she failed to think about what might happen to her as a widow, including what steps she could take to survive her loss emotionally. Because she relied on a close circle of married friends, she had to deal with the reality of being an outsider after her husband's death or, as she put it, a "fifth wheel." This is common. While her husband was alive, Luann could have prevented that situation by going back to school or joining organizations that would have put her in contact with people of different ages and circumstances: married, divorced, widowed, young, old. *It's what all women should be doing—planning and preparing to thrive independently and happily no matter what happens.*

With such planning, Luann would have broadened the circle of friends she could rely on for the social and emotional support she needs. Because Luann finds it depressing to be around old people much of the time, this strategy would have helped her find the diversity of friends she needed when tragedy struck. Someone in this mix of people might even have been a special someone with whom she could later share her unforeseen widowhood.

The "He's Too Young for Me" Trap

There is one last caution that I want to give you, and it is directly related to Luanne's situation. All too often, the "I'm too old" attitude affects your decisions about relationships. What I'm talking about here is the stigma, even in our "enlightened" society, still attached to an older woman dating a younger man. I call it the "He's too young for me" trap, and it is something that you want to think about if you find yourself suddenly looking for a new partner to share the rest of your life with.

We all know how acceptable it is in our culture for an older man to marry a much younger woman. People may raise their eyebrows, but because it's so common we let it pass and think that she did it for the money and isn't he the lucky duck. However, we're not nearly so forgiving if an older woman marries or even dates a younger man. Old ladies are supposed to be with old men, right? I've seen lonely, older widowed women go to ridiculous lengths to get the attention of the most eligible (and that ain't saying much) old geezer at the senior center. It's sad how fierce the competition can be. (I saw this bizarre behavior while on the job, and it was one of the things that motivated me to avoid the Senior Culture Club.) The "He's too young for me" trap is simply this: you succumb to the notion that if you marry or date a younger man, you are a "cradle robber." It's one of the more insidious forms of sexism and ageism, if you think about it.

But let's face it. If you've taken care of yourself both mentally and physically, you as an "older woman" can be a great catch for a younger man. The reasons are too numerous to mention. (But you do know what those reasons are, don't you? Hint: older women can cook—in more ways than one.) An older guy is generally not a great catch (and you do know why not, right?). Approximately 30 percent of men age sixty and older are estimated to have low testosterone. This condition is often accompanied by low bone and muscle mass, increased fat mass, low energy, and impaired physical, sexual, and cognitive functions. (See "Study: Low Testosterone Levels May Increase Risk of Death in Older Men" at www.foxnews.com/story/0,2933,301940,00.html.)

Who wants a broken down, cantankerous old geezer? The good news is that symptoms that accompany low testosterone can be addressed with carefully adjusted hormone replacement. Unfortunately for men, it's not as acceptable to seek treatment for hormone deficiency as it is for women. It is also unfortunate that many traditional physicians are wary of testosterone replacement therapy. However, if around age forty men were tested and given appropriate hormone replacement, many could stay healthy and vital far longer. There would be fewer grumpy, incapacitated old guys, to the delight of many older women.

All nudging and winking aside, statistics show that women tend to live longer than men and that a woman over forty marrying a younger man is more likely to have a mate whose life span matches her own.

While it's impossible to say where any stigma originates, the "He's too young for me" mentality probably has something to do with the cultural norms of how women marry when they're young. In the days of arranged marriages, it was quite common for a teenaged daughter to be given to a man twenty years her senior. The much older man had a better dowry—in other words, he could pay more for the young flesh. Now that most of us marry for love and not because of what our parents want, the age discrepancy has lessened; however, the cultural norm has remained. Now, when a woman in her twenties marries, it's usually to a man five to ten years older. That still makes sense because it takes so long for men to mature.

Unfortunately, not too many of these young woman–older man marriages last forever anymore. Most of them aren't committed to riding off into the sunset together for better or worse. By age forty, if not sooner, they are searching once more for the perfect partner.

An older woman has a choice. If she is forty or older and looking for a partner, it doesn't make sense for her to look for someone too much older. It may be okay if she is forty and he is fifty—for a while. However, if they stay together when she is sixty-five and he is seventy-five, her chances of becoming a caretaker instead a wife are significant. (That may not be considered a burden if the couple has been together since their youth and has enjoyed a good relationship.) So are her chances of becoming a widow. That's worth thinking about, which our culture doesn't want to do.

So what about Luann's dilemma? The smartest thing that she could do is start taking care of herself, both mentally and physically, and then start looking for a new love. She can help this along by telling all her friends, married and single, that she's looking for the right companion—and he can definitely be younger! Oh, and one more thing: if she limits her socializing to women friends, the chances of her finding a partner diminish greatly.

It's never easy to think about losing your life partner. We all would like to think that we'll go together. But the reality says something different, and the financial and emotional drain can be so great that it's important to at least think about. If you're brave, plan it out on paper.

So, if you do happen to find yourself in a situation where you want to find another life partner to live out your days with, don't be afraid. If you're a mature woman, it's perfectly acceptable to have a relationship with a younger man if it makes you happy, it isn't illegal, and it doesn't cast doubt on your sanity. Don't be deterred if people raise their eyebrows or make snide remarks. Know that those who tsk-tsk your good fortune secretly wish they had the guts (or were lucky enough) to do the same. If I were a forty-something woman like Demi Moore, I might hesitate to date or marry twenty-something Ashton Kutcher, but I'm not going to tsk-tsk her good fortune—and more importantly, *his* good fortune! Good for the both of them!

Women who date or marry younger men never become Little Old Ladies!

Celebrate the Payoff: Three Major Advantages to Aging Agelessly

If you learn how to control and manage the aging process early in your life—if you plan well—then the benefits become too numerous to mention. The payoff comes when you are old in years but not in mind or spirit. Unfortunately, you don't get to experience and appreciate the payoff until you're actually "there." I am "there," so I can tell you that planning and pit-bull determination reap incredible benefits.

What's the most important benefit of aging agelessly? After all is said and done, it comes down to having freedom and independence and being in a state of constant growth and productivity.

Freedom is a gift that few elderly or old people enjoy because when they were younger they didn't plan for the kind of life they wanted in later years. They were without vision. They didn't manage the youthful gifts they had been given. They just allowed life to happen, which means they aged traditionally.

Certainly, even with the best of plans, life has a way of throwing a wild pitch when you least expect it. But in spite of that, if you work diligently and prepare, if you develop an inner toughness, if you unleash your innate pit-bull survival instinct, you can even deal with unexpected health issues effectively.

If you doubt the importance of having freedom in your later years, know that the *one thing* old people fear the most (besides not having enough money) is loss of freedom and independence. They don't want to end their days in a nursing home or be dependent on others. Yet, when you don't prepare well early on, that outcome can be anticipated.

Here, concisely, is the prize won by the person who ages agelessly:

- **Freedom from fear:** If you stay healthy and strong physically and mentally, your chances of becoming a victim of financial, physical, or mental elder abuse decrease significantly. Perpetrators prey only on those perceived to be weak and vulnerable.

- **Independence and self-determination:** If at age eighty-five and beyond you are strong physically and mentally, you can live with the same independence as you did twenty-five or more years earlier. You can enjoy a vibrant second life that few attain but many envy. You won't have to wait for someone else to take you where you want to go or tell you what to do. With carefully nurtured good health, you can live with joyful abandon. Because you stay productive, you can be a generous giver rather than a needy taker.

- **Opportunities for growth:** If you have remained healthy and strong physically and mentally, you can continue to grow, produce, and prosper financially. You can successfully avoid the decline-oriented Senior Culture Club. You can be a mentor and role model for younger people, go back to school, or even start a new business. You can cultivate new relationships. The sky is the limit when you learn and implement the fifteen strategies offered in this book.

Living in healthy, productive, energized, joyful freedom in advanced age is the prize you win when you learn to use the fifteen strategies well before you reach "old age." It is the ultimate program to avoid becoming a Little Old Lady. It works for me, and it will work for you. Start today to create the future of your choice!

Apply All You've Learned Right Away

Here is a summary of what I hope you've learned through reading this book.

- You have learned proven, author tried and tested, strategies to achieve ageless aging and to avoid becoming a Little Old Lady.

- You know more about the senior culture mentality and why it contributes to premature decline more than anything else, and you know how you can avoid becoming part of it.

- You've been told to stay in charge of what goes on in your head because that's where decline originates— not with the passage of time.

- You've learned why it's important to choose not to have "senior moments."

- You've discovered my ultimate power tool to control the aging process, something not found (to my knowledge) in other antiaging books.

- You now know how to manage your mental and physical capacity—because without a strong, healthy, flexible mind and body, you will age traditionally.

- You are now aware that you can choose to control your existence manager, which is designed to take you to the end of your life on its terms, not on yours.

- You have discovered your fierce "inner pit bull" that you can train to help you manage your aging process.

- You've been challenged to eliminate outdated traditions and cultural norms that are mired in the Stone Age.

- You've been made aware of the outcome of choosing to "age gracefully."

- You've been encouraged to adopt new stages of aging that will help you stay youthful and productive longer.

- You've learned to protect and use your life force—that nebulous energy and power that only young people appear to have.

- You know the importance of understanding that to overcome decline, attitude is everything. You've heard that before, but everyone needs a constant reminder and help doing it.

- You've learned to understand the consequences of telling your age and dwelling on the significance of your chronological age.

- You've internalized the importance of taking care of your health and how best to do it.

- You've been made aware of the power of group dependence and consensus thinking and how it can derail your desire to age agelessly—*and* how to avoid or manage it.

• You are now better prepared for losing a loved one at a critical time of your life.

• You have been given helpful links in the resources section of this book to access additional information.

Meet the Author

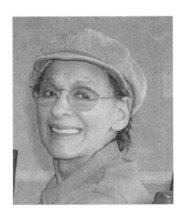

Barbara Morris, 79

Current photo

*Aging Agelessly —
Living Agelessly*

Barbara Morris is a pharmacist, writer, motivational speaker, and antiaging expert. She is the author of *Put Old on Hold* and publishes a monthly newsletter. She has appeared on TV and before enthusiastic audiences across the country. Her expertise has been cited in Art Linkletter and Mark Victor Hansen's book, *How to Make the Rest of Your Life the Best of Your Life*. Her website is www.PutOldonHold.com.

Resources

This list is a starting place for information only; it is not a source of medical advice. Consult a physician for competent medical advice. To avoid overwhelming newbies, I haven't included every excellent book, magazine, and website that I use. As with any reading you do, use judgment and discernment in evaluating worthiness. All web links were working at time of publication.

Books

How to Make the Rest of Your Life the Best of Your Life
by Mark Victor Hansen and Art Linkletter

Smart Drugs II (Smart Drug Series, Volume 2)
by Ward Dean

Normal Blood Test Scores Aren't Good Enough!
by Ellie Cullen, Ann Louise Gittleman, and Betty Kamen

(Most alternative physicians rely on comprehensive blood tests to evaluate patient health.)

Your Body's Many Cries for Water
by Fereydoon Batmanghelidj, MD

The Miracle of Bio-Identical Hormones, 2nd edition
by Michael E. Platt, MD

Lipitor: Thief of Memory
by Duane Graveline, MD; Jay S. Cohen; and Kilmer S. McCully

Fast Food Nation
by Eric Schlosser

Fast Food Nation Tie-in: The Dark Side of the All-American Meal (P.S.)
by Eric Schlosser

The pH Miracle: Balance Your Diet, Reclaim Your Health
by Robert O. Young and Shelley Redford Young

The Perricone Prescription
by Nicholas Perricone, MD

The Perricone Promise
by Nicolas Perricone, MD

Fantastic Voyage: Live Long Enough to Live Forever
by Ray Kurzweil

Don't Stop the Career Clock: Rejecting the Myths of Aging for a New Way to Work in the 21st Century
by Helen Harkness, PhD

Bold Retirement: Mining Your Own Silver for a Rich Life
By Mary Lloyd

Drug-Induced Nutrient Depletion Handbook
by Ross Pelton, PhD; James B. LaValle; Ernest B. Hawkins; and Daniel L. Krinsky

Successful Aging
by John Wallis Rowe, MD, and Robert L. Kahn

The Antioxidant Miracle: Put Lipoic Acid, Pycnogenol, and Vitamins E and C to Work for You
by Lester Packer and Carol Colman

Cosmetic Surgery: Before, Between, and After
by Susan Gail

Over 40 and Gettin' Stronger
by Phyllis Rogers

Put Old on Hold
by Barbara Morris, RPh.

No Sweat? Know Sweat! The Definitive Guide to Reclaim Your Health
by Bill Akpinar, MD, DDS, DrAc, PhD

Bless Your Stress
by C. Leslie Charles and Mimi Donaldson

Newsletters, Magazines, Websites
(Click on the main site, and navigate to the desired area.)

Life Extension magazine: www.lef.org/magazine

Julian Whitaker, MD (print newsletter):
www.drwhitaker.com

Stephen Sinatra, MD (print newsletter):
www.drsinatra.com

Joseph Mercola, DO (website): www.mercola.com

Miscellaneous

Wyeth Report
"New study finds increased multivitamin use by the elderly could save Medicare $1.6 billion" http://putoldonhold.net/Lewin%20Report.pdf

Resources for Blood Tests

www.YourFutureHealth.com

Life Extension Foundation: www.lef.org

Antiaging Physician Locator

American College for Advancement of Medicine:
www.acam.org

American Academy of Anti-Aging Medicine (A4M): www.worldhealth.net

Alzheimer's Disease Research

This is just a sampling of evidence that Alzheimer's disease and normal cognitive decline may be more preventable than now believed:

Sugary drinks linked to Alzheimer's, says study:
www.nutraingredients.com/news/printNewsBis. asp?id=81927

Pomegranate juice may cut Alzheimer's risk:
www.nutraingredients.com/news/ng.asp?n=70982&m=1 NIEO03&c=nszedopdfzvbmwd

Green tea could protect against Alzheimer's:
www.ap-foodtechnology.com/news/ng.asp?n=66142&m= 2APF308&c=nszedopdfzvbmwd

Med schools failing on nutrition teaching:
www.nutraingredients-usa.com/news/ng.asp?n=67000& m=1NIU412&c=nszedopdfzvbmwd

Red Wine again linked to slowing Alzheimer's:
www.nutraingredients-usa.com/news/ng.asp?n=70901& m=2FSNO10&idP=5&c=nszedopdfzvbmwd

Antioxidant, polyphenol-rich Med diet could slash Alzheimer's risk: www.nutraingredients.com/news/ng.a sp?n=71194&m=2FSNO25&idP=2&c=nszedopdfzvbmwd

Curcumin could cut plaque build-up linked to Alzheimer's: www.nutraingredients.com/news/ng.asp?n =71039&m=2FSNO10&idP=2&c=nszedopdfzvbmwd

Fruit and veg juice may reduce Alzheimer's risk: www. nutraingredients.com/news/ng.asp?n=70233&m=2NIEO3 0&c=nszedopdfzvbmwd&test=1

Omega-3s show promise for very mild Alzheimer's: www.nutraingredients.com/news/ng.asp?n=71152&m=2F SNO10&idP=2&c=nszedopdfzvbmwd

Vitamin E-rich vegetables could slow cognitive decline: www.nutraingredients.com/news/ng.asp?n=71520&m=2 NIEO30&c=nszedopdfzvbmwd&test=1

Omega fatty acids to stop mental decline, says study: www.nutraingredients-usa.com/news/ng.asp?n=71726& m=1NIUO31&c=nszedopdfzvbmwd

Bonus Gift!

I've given you my *No More Little Old Ladies!* strategies, and as a bonus for purchasing this book, you get a *free* workbook (a forty-seven-dollar value)! Knowing how to do something and actually doing it are two separate things. The workbook helps you develop the right mind-set and lifestyle and will motivate you to prepare now for what lies ahead.

Go to your computer, and enter this link in your web browser:

www.agelessaging.net/lol_workbook_request.html

It will bring up a page with a form on it. Fill in the form to confirm your request, and you will receive the link to the workbook right away.

Antiaging Coaching
Available

Want to avoid becoming a Little Old Lady but don't know where to start or what to do? Barbara is coaching a limited number of students. For more information, visit:

www.agelessaging.net/coaching

Questions? Comments? Suggestions?

Contact Barbara at ageless.aging@gmail.com.

BUY A SHARE OF THE FUTURE IN YOUR COMMUNITY

These certificates make great holiday, graduation and birthday gifts that can be personalized with the recipient's name. The cost of one S.H.A.R.E. or one square foot is $54.17. The personalized certificate is suitable for framing and will state the number of shares purchased and the amount of each share, as well as the recipient's name. The home that you participate in "building" will last for many years and will continue to grow in value.

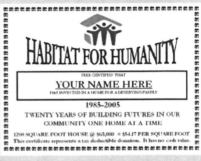

Here is a sample SHARE certificate:

THIS CERTIFIES THAT

YOUR NAME HERE

HAS INVESTED IN A HOME FOR A DESERVING FAMILY

1985-2005

TWENTY YEARS OF BUILDING FUTURES IN OUR COMMUNITY ONE HOME AT A TIME

1200 SQUARE FOOT HOUSE @ $65,000 = $54.17 PER SQUARE FOOT
This certificate represents a tax deductible donation. It has no cash value.

YES, I WOULD LIKE TO HELP!

*I support the work that Habitat for Humanity does and I want to be part of the excitement! As a donor, I will receive periodic updates on your construction activities but, more importantly, I know my gift will help a family in our community realize the dream of homeownership. **I would like to SHARE in your efforts against substandard housing in my community!** (Please print below)*

PLEASE SEND ME _____ SHARES at $54.17 EACH = $ $_____

In Honor Of: _____

Occasion: (Circle One)   HOLIDAY   BIRTHDAY   ANNIVERSARY

      OTHER: _____

Address of Recipient: _____

Gift From: _____ *Donor Address:* _____

Donor Email: _____

I AM ENCLOSING A CHECK FOR $ $_____ PAYABLE TO HABITAT FOR HUMANITY <u>OR</u> PLEASE CHARGE MY VISA OR MASTERCARD *(CIRCLE ONE)*

Card Number _____ Expiration Date: _____

Name as it appears on Credit Card _____ Charge Amount $ _____

Signature _____

Billing Address _____

Telephone # Day _____ Eve _____

PLEASE NOTE: Your contribution is tax-deductible to the fullest extent allowed by law.
Habitat for Humanity • P.O. Box 1443 • Newport News, VA 23601 • 757-596-5553
www.HelpHabitatforHumanity.org

MAY   2010

LaVergne, TN USA
28 April 2010
180883LV00001B/25/P

9 781600 375217